Practical
Handbook of
Oral Pathology

Practical
Handbook of
Oral Pathology

Arush Thakur MDS
Ex-Assistant Professor
Department of Oral Pathology and Microbiology
Government Dental College and Hospital, Mumbai

Jagdish Vishnu Tupkari MDS
Ex-Dean, Ex-Professor and Head
Department of Oral Pathology and Microbiology
Government Dental College and Hospital, Mumbai

Tabita Joy Chettiankandy (Benjamin) MDS
Professor (Academic) and Head
Department of Oral Pathology and Microbiology
Government Dental College and Hospital, Mumbai

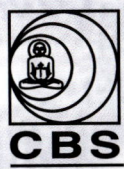

CBS

CBS Publishers & Distributors Pvt Ltd

New Delhi • Bengaluru • Chennai • Kochi • Kolkata • Mumbai
Hyderabad • Jharkhand • Nagpur • Patna • Pune • Uttarakhand

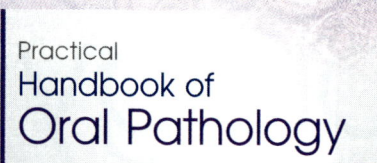

Practical
Handbook of
Oral Pathology

ISBN: 978-93-89688-48-1

Copyright © Authors and Publisher

First Edition: 2021

Published by Satish Kumar Jain and produced by Varun Jain for

CBS Publishers & Distributors Pvt Ltd

4819/XI Prahlad Street, 24 Ansari Road, Daryaganj, New Delhi 110 002, India.
Ph: 23289259, 23266861, 23266867 Website: www.cbspd.com
Fax: 011-23243014   e-mail: delhi@cbspd.com; cbspubs@airtelmail.in.

Corporate Office: 204 FIE, Industrial Area, Patparganj, Delhi 110 092
Ph: 4934 4934   Fax: 4934 4935   e-mail: publishing@cbspd.com; publicity@cbspd.com

Branches

- **Bengaluru:** Seema House 2975, 17th Cross, K.R. Road, Banasankari 2nd Stage, Bengaluru 560 070, Karnataka
  Ph: +91-80-26771678/79   Fax: +91-80-26771680   e-mail: bangalore@cbspd.com
- **Chennai:** 7, Subbaraya Street, Shenoy Nagar, Chennai 600 030, Tamil Nadu
  Ph: +91-44-26680620/26681266   Fax: +91-44-42032115   e-mail: chennai@cbspd.com
- **Kochi:** 42/1325, 1326, Power House Road, Opp KSEB, Power House, Ernakulam 682 018, Kochi, Kerala
  Ph: +91-484-4059061-65   Fax: +91-484-4059065   e-mail: kochi@cbspd.com
- **Kolkata:** 6/B, Ground Floor, Rameswar Shaw Road, Kolkata-700 014, West Bengal
  Ph: +91-33-22891126, 22891127, 22891128   e-mail: kolkata@cbspd.com
- **Mumbai:** 83-C, Dr E Moses Road, Worli, Mumbai-400018, Maharashtra
  Ph: +91-22-24902340/41   Fax: +91-22-24902342   e-mail: mumbai@cbspd.com

Representatives

• **Hyderabad**	0-9885175004	• **Jharkhand**	0-9811541605	• **Nagpur**	0-9421945513
• **Patna**	0-9334159340	• **Pune**	0-9623451994	• **Uttarakhand**	0-9716462459

Printed At : Goyal Offset Works (P) Limited

to
my parents and brother

Foreword

It is an honour and privilege to have been asked to write the Foreword to the book entitled *Practical Handbook of Oral Pathology* for 3rd year BDS written with great efforts by Dr Arush Thakur along with valuable contributions and guidance of co-authors Dr JV Tupkari and Dr Tabita Joy.

I have known Dr Arush Thakur as a hard-working and sincere postgraduate student and the dedicated lecturer keen to impart knowledge to the students, and also a desire to learn, understand and apply the knowledge for patient services.

This book is written taking into consideration the 3rd year undergraduate students and emphasis is given to the practical part of oral pathology. This book will help the students in understanding the histopathological aspects of lesions affecting the oral and maxillofacial region along with important, point-wise details of clinical features. The description of slides is given in very informative and in a 'students-friendly' language, which will definitely help the students not only to gain practical knowledge but also face the examination with greater confidence. Another important aspect of this book is the *viva voce* questions which are given at the end of this book.

I personally feel that this book is excellent and will be of profound help to the students to understand the microscopic features of oral and maxillofacial lesions.

With regards and best wishes.

Dr HR Umarji
Ex-Professor and Head
Department of Oral Medicine and Radiology
Government Dental College and Hospital
Mumbai, Maharashtra, India

Preface

Practical Handbook of Oral Pathology for 3rd BDS is primarily written for 3rd year undergraduate students of dental faculty. The basic idea for writing this book came during my interactions with 3rd year undergraduates during my postgraduate days. These interactions helped me to comprehend their difficulties in understanding the histopathological slides. The motive behind this venture is to help students with understanding of the basic slides along with intricacies of viva voce questions.

I would make no claim regarding the originality of text written in the book. The information related to the different oral lesions is concised and simplified. The histopathological photographs include herewith are all stained with hematoxylin and eosin stain.

During my tenure as a postgraduate, I had the privilege of learning oral pathology under the guidance of Dr Jagdish Vishnu Tupkari, Ex-Dean, Ex-Professor and Head, Department of Oral Pathology, Government Dental College and Hospital, Mumbai. I am very grateful to my guide Tupkari sir for patiently listening to my ideas and giving his unbiased opinion all the time. I also want to thank him for helping and allowing me to go ahead with my notion in completing and publishing this book.

I also want to thank Dr Tabita Joy (co-author) for her constant support and guidance during the write up of this book.

I am extremely grateful to Dr Manisha Sardar, Dr Pooja Siwach, Dr Amrut Hanchate, Dr Sayali Jhadav, Dr Anuradha, Dr Rashmi, Dr Ruchika Aggarwal, Dr Zaneta and PG students for all the, motivation.

I consider myself blessed to be a part of Government Dental College and Hospital, Mumbai.

I am also thankful to CBS Publishers & Distributors. I would like to put on record the sincere efforts of Mr YN Arjuna (Senior Vice President Publishing, Editorial and Publicity), and his team comprising Ms Ritu Chawla (GM Production), Mr Parmod Kumar (DTP Operator), and Mr Sanjay Chauhan (Graphic Designer), for bringing out the book in the present form.

Arush Thakur

Contents

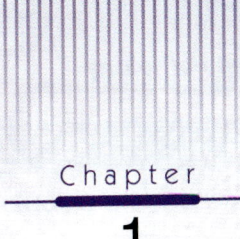
Odontogenic Cysts

ODONTOGENIC CYST

CYST: Kramer (1974) has defined a cyst as 'a pathological cavity having fluid, semifluid or gaseous contents and which is not created by the accumulation of pus'. Most cysts, but not all, are lined by epithelium.

Histopathologically almost all cystic lesions (true cyst) show cystic lumen, lining epithelium and connective tissue wall. While making the diagnosis of any cystic lesion, content of cystic lumen, configuration of lining epithelium and cystic wall should be taken into consideration.

Most cysts, but not all, are lined by epithelium.

ODONTOGENIC CYSTS HAVE BEEN BROADLY CLASSIFIED BASED

- On the presence or absence of epithelial lining.
- On their location as cysts of the jaws cysts of the maxillary antrum and cysts of the soft tissues of mouth face and neck.
- On origin as odontogenic non-odontogenic, developmental, inflammatory traumatic, and parasitic cysts.

The World Health Organization has classifed the cysts of the jaws first in 1970, later 1992, then 2005 and recently in 2017.

We have enumerated a few commonly occurring cysts which are based on the epidemiological studies on cysts of the orofacial region in India.

1. Odontogenic keratocyst
2. Dentigerous cyst
3. Radicular cyst
4. Residual cyst
5. Glandular odontogenic cyst
6. Lateral periodontal cyst
7. Mucous extravasation cyst
8. Mucous retention cyst
9. Traumatic bone cyst
10. Aneurysmal cyst
11. Parasitic cyst

ODONTOGENIC CYST (DEVELOPMENTAL)

Odontogenic Keratocyst (OKC)/Keratocystic Odontogenic Tumor (KCOT)

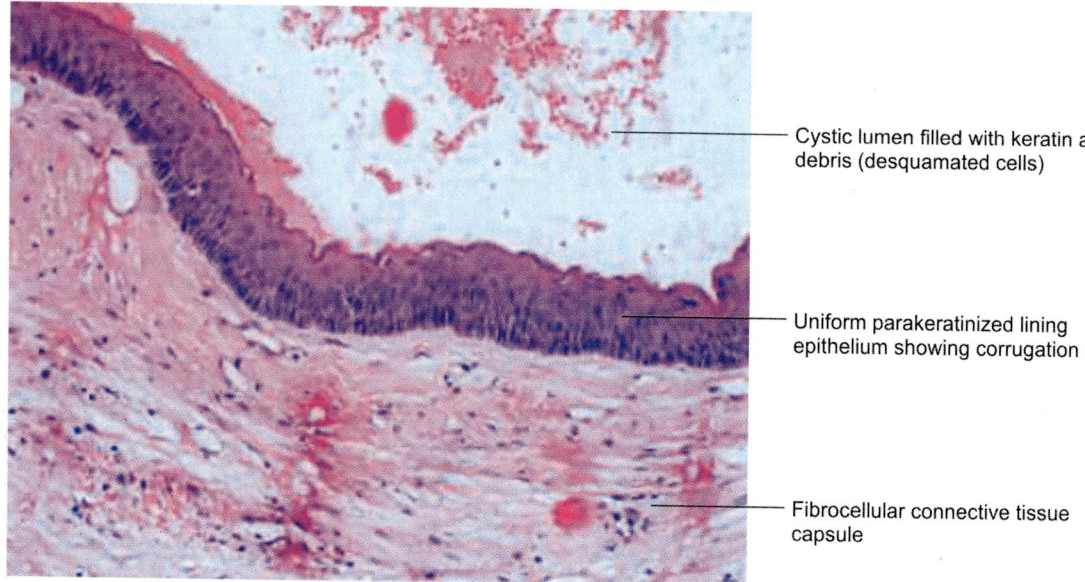

Cystic lumen filled with keratin and debris (desquamated cells)

Uniform parakeratinized lining epithelium showing corrugation

Fibrocellular connective tissue capsule

Fig. 1.1: 10X

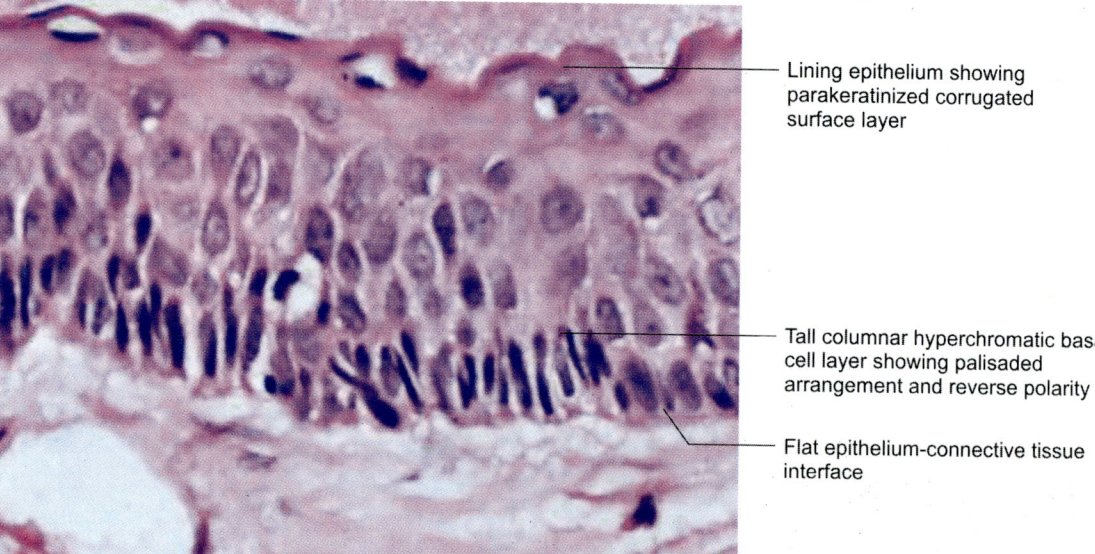

Lining epithelium showing parakeratinized corrugated surface layer

Tall columnar hyperchromatic basal cell layer showing palisaded arrangement and reverse polarity

Flat epithelium-connective tissue interface

Fig. 1.2: 40X

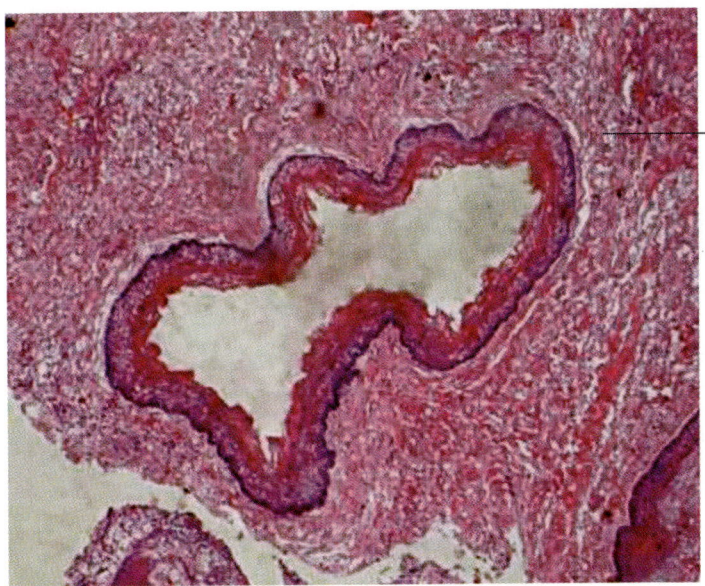

Daughter cyst in the connective tissue capsule

Fig. 1.3: 10X

Odontogenic Keratocyst (OKC/KCOT)

Key Points

- Developmental odontogenic cyst.
- Posterior region of mandible (body and ramus regions) most common site.
- Predominantly occurs in second and third decade.
- Frequently occurs in males compared to females.
- Associated with nevoid basal cell carcinoma syndrome (NBCCS).
- More aggressive biological behaviour than orthokeratinized odontogenic cyst (OOC).
- Radiographically: Usually shows a well-defined unilocular radiolucent lesion, but can also be multilocular with scalloping border.
- Clinically and radiographically OKC commonly mimics unicystic ameloblastoma, dentigerous cyst.
- It is named keratocyst, because of the extensive keratin produced by the cystic lining that fills the cystic lumen.
- Cystic fluid has protein below 3.5 g per 100 ml.
- Cystic fluid varies straw coloured to thicker creamy material depending upon the amount of keratin present.

Histopathological Picture

Histopathologically, OKC Usually Shows Classical Picture

- Parakeratinized, stratified, squamous lining epithelium.
- 5–8 cell layers thick cystic lining.
- Corrugated parakeratin surface layer.
- Palisaded, basophilic columnar basal cell layer.
- Epithelium connective tissue interface is flat.
- Connective tissue shows daughter cyst occasionally.
- Connective tissue capsule is loose fibrocellular with parallelly arranged collagen fibers.

Additional Point

The World Health Organization in 2005 had reclassified and renamed the odontogenic keratocyst as keratocystic odontogenic tumor, an odontogenic tumor derived from the odontogenic epithelium, but later in 2017 again renamed it as odontogenic keratocyst and placed it back in cyst category. (Controversial nature)

ORTHOKERATINIZED ODONTOGENIC CYST (OOC)

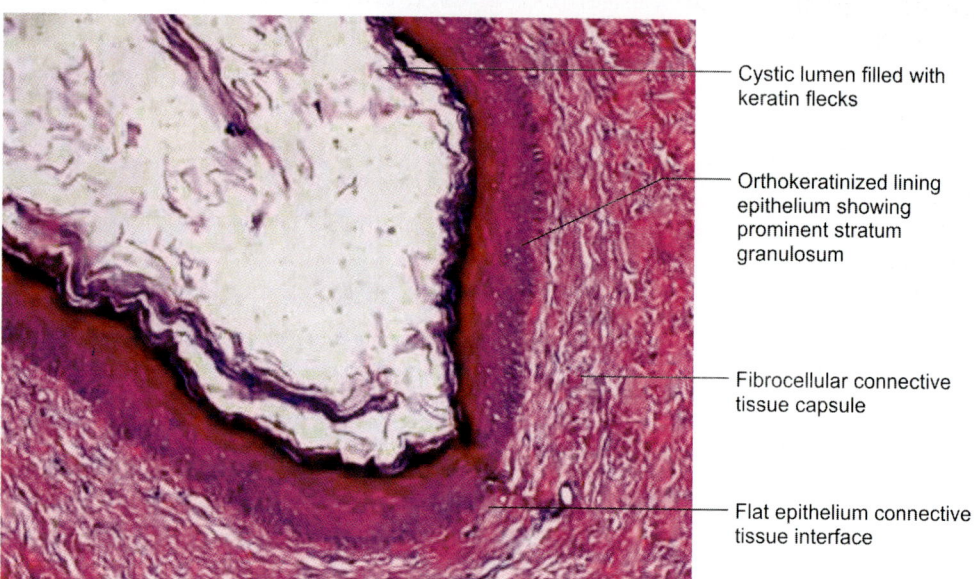

Cystic lumen filled with keratin flecks

Orthokeratinized lining epithelium showing prominent stratum granulosum

Fibrocellular connective tissue capsule

Flat epithelium connective tissue interface

Fig. 1.4: 10X

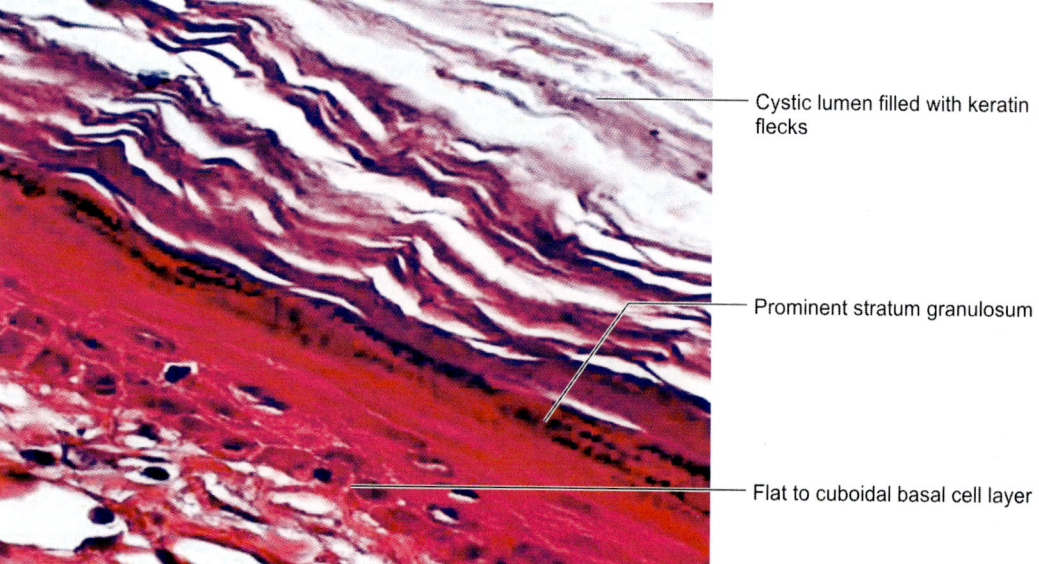

Cystic lumen filled with keratin flecks

Prominent stratum granulosum

Flat to cuboidal basal cell layer

Fig. 1.5: 40X

Key Points

- Developmental odontogenic cyst, considered as a variant of the OKC.
- Mandible is more affected than maxilla usually involving the molar-ramus region.
- Predilection for the third and the fourth decade.
- OOC occurs more frequently in males than in females.
- Radiographically, most of the cases appear as unilocular lesion with well-defined margins.
- The lesions with similar clinical and radiographic presentation should be considered in the differential diagnosis such as dentigerous cyst, OKC, ameloblastoma in particular unicystic ameloblastoma (cystic variant of ameloblastoma).

Histopathological Picture

- Histologically OOC shows a cystic cavity filled with and flecks.
- Cystic cavity is lined by an orthokeratinized epithelium of varying thickness with thick keratinization, displaying a well-developed stratum granulosum and a well-defined flat or low cuboidal basal cell layer.
- Basal cells show no tendency to palisade, neither nuclear polarization nor hyperchromatism.
- A hypocellular spinous cell layer is usually made-up of polyhedral to flattened cells with eosinophilic cytoplasm.
- Epithelium connective tissue interface is flat.
- Flat to cuboidal basal cell layer.

DENTIGEROUS CYST

Cystic lumen

Thin non-keratinized lining epithelium 2–4 cell layer in thickness with flat epithelium connective tissue interface

Connective tissue wall is loose resembling embryonal tissue

Fig. 1.6: 4X

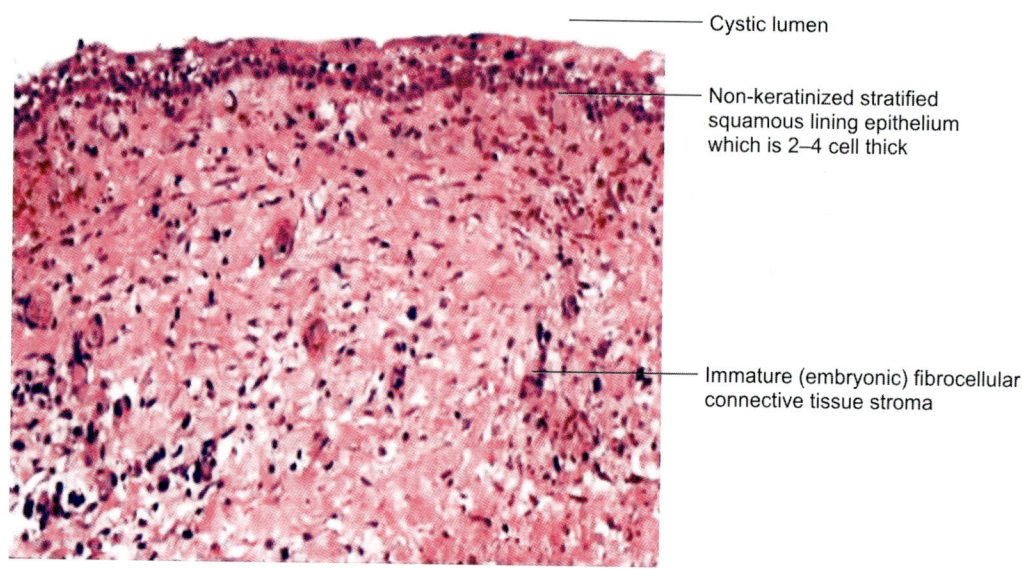

Cystic lumen

Non-keratinized stratified squamous lining epithelium which is 2–4 cell thick

Immature (embryonic) fibrocellular connective tissue stroma

Fig. 1.7: 10X

Key Points

- Developmental odontogenic cyst associated with impacted tooth.
- It may be found enclosing a complex compound odontoma or involving a supernumerary tooth.
- Most of the lesion associated with mandibular and maxillary 3rd molars.
- Predilection in second and third decade.
- Slight male predominance.
- Bilateral and multiple cysts are usually found in association with a number of syndromes including Cleidocranial dysplasia and Maroteaux-Lamy syndrome.

Radiographically

Radiolucent area usually associated with an unerupted tooth crown.

- Dentigerous cyst can be suspected when the space is >5 mm (normal follicular space is 3–4 mm).
- Radiological variations of the dentigerous cyst: Central, lateral or circumferential type.
- The dentigerous cyst is usually a unilocular lesion, but occasionally multilocular appearance may be seen.

Histopathological Picture

- Cyst lining resembles reduced enamel epithelium.
- Connective tissue wall is of embryonal type consisting of loosely arranged collagen fibers.
- An additional finding, is the presence of Rushton bodies within the lining epithelium, especially in inflamed cyst. These are peculiar linear, often curved, hyaline bodies with variable stainability which are of uncertain origin, questionable nature and unknown significance.
- In case of inflamed dentigerous cyst one can find proliferative lining epithelium with rete peg formation, connective tissue wall which is more collagenized (mature) with inflammatory cells.

Additional Points

- Aspirated cystic fluid is usually thin, watery yellow colored and occasionally blood tinged.
- Ameloblastoma may develop from cystic lining or from odontogenic rest present in the cystic wall.
- Epidermoid carcinoma may arise from the lining epithelium.
- Mucoepidermoid carcinoma can also develop from the cystic lining.

RADICULAR CYST

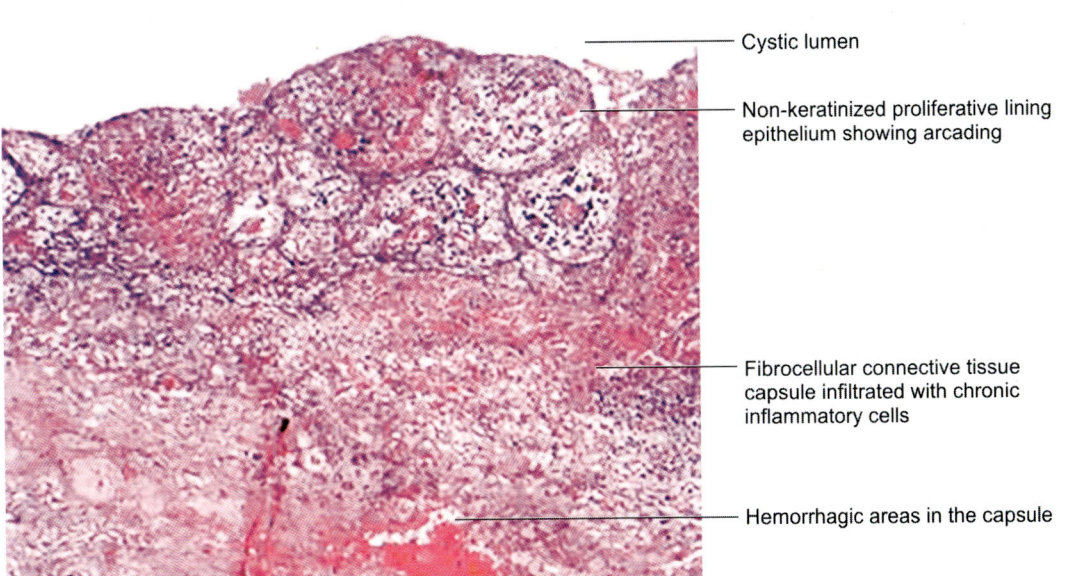

Cystic lumen

Non-keratinized proliferative lining epithelium showing arcading

Fibrocellular connective tissue capsule infiltrated with chronic inflammatory cells

Hemorrhagic areas in the capsule

Fig. 1.8: 4X

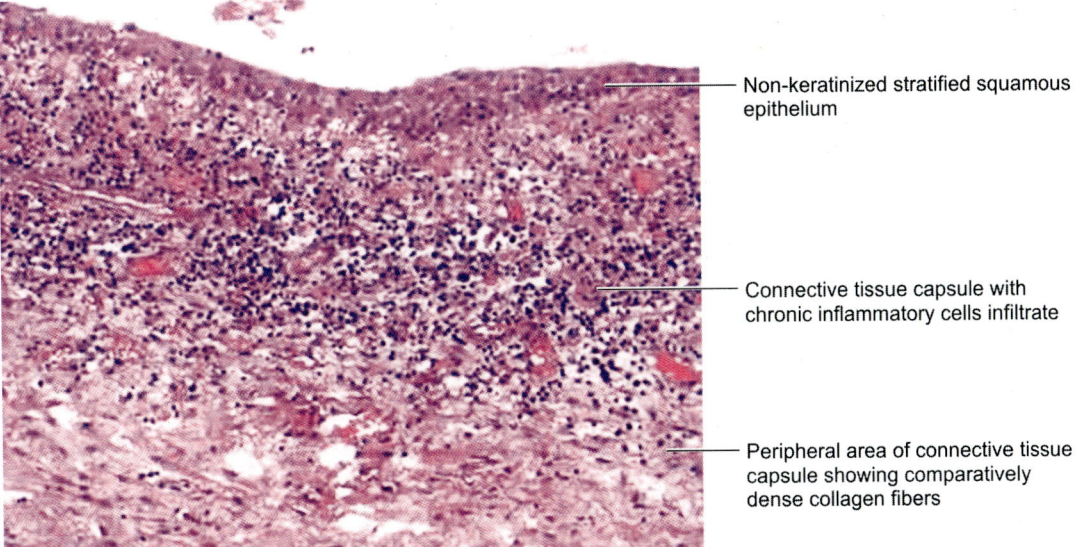

Non-keratinized stratified squamous epithelium

Connective tissue capsule with chronic inflammatory cells infiltrate

Peripheral area of connective tissue capsule showing comparatively dense collagen fibers

Fig. 1.9: 10X

Radicular Cyst/Periapical Cyst

Key Points

- Inflammatory odontogenic cyst.
- Always associated with non-vital tooth.
- After removal of an associated tooth the cyst which remains is called residual cyst.
- Maxillary anterior region most common site.
- Male predominance.

Radiographically

Usually shows a well-defined unilocular radiolucent lesion with scalloping.

Histopathological Picture

Histopathologically, radicular cyst shows:

- Usually non-keratinized stratified, squamous epithelium which can be 1 to 100 cell layer in thickness.
- Epithelium shows proliferation, spongiosis and arcading.
- Connective tissue capsule is infiltrated with inflammatory cell infiltrate.
- Depending upon distance from lumen and duration of cyst the fiber arrangement and size varies.
- Rushton bodies, composed of an eosinophilic material resembling hyalinized collagen.
- These are peculiar linear, often curved, hyaline bodies with variable stainability which are of uncertain origin, questionable nature and unknown significance.

Additional Point

Aspiration biopsy reveals cholesterol crystals with macrophages (granular cells) resembling blueprint of house under the light microscope.

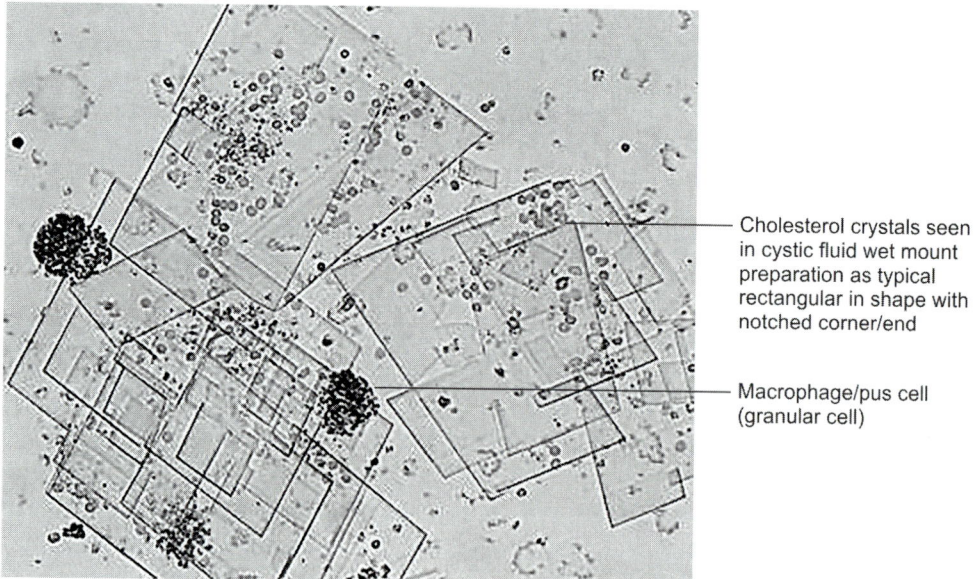

Cholesterol crystals seen in cystic fluid wet mount preparation as typical rectangular in shape with notched corner/end

Macrophage/pus cell (granular cell)

Fig. 1.10: 10X

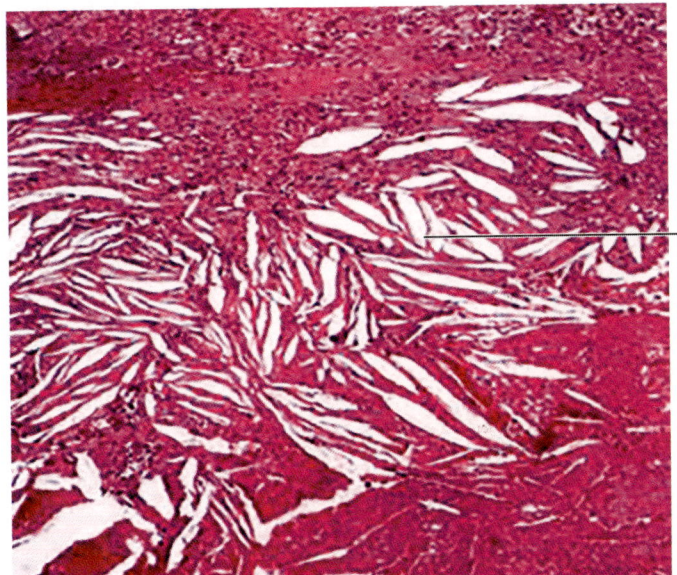

Numerous cholesterol clefts formed after removal of cholesterol crystals during tissue processing

Fig. 1.11: 10X cholesterol clefts

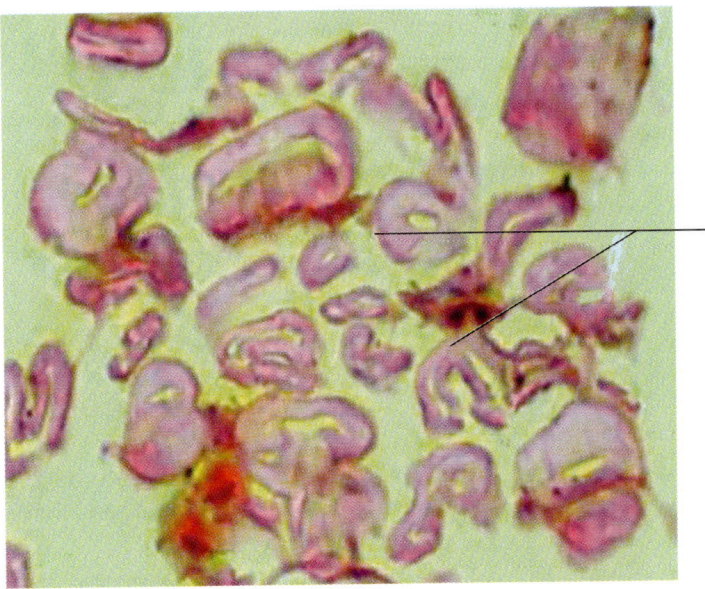

Numerous Rushton bodies

Fig. 1.12: 10X Rushton bodies

CALCIFYING ODONTOGENIC CYST (COC)

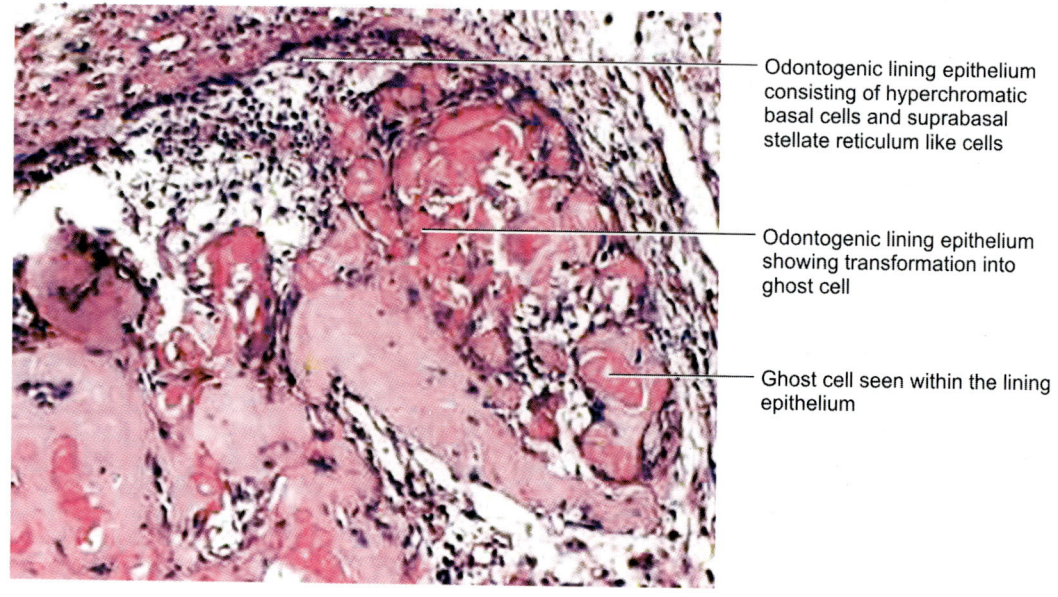

Odontogenic lining epithelium consisting of hyperchromatic basal cells and suprabasal stellate reticulum like cells

Odontogenic lining epithelium showing transformation into ghost cell

Ghost cell seen within the lining epithelium

Fig. 1.13: 10X

Key Points

- Also known as 'keratinizing and calcifying odontogenic cyst', Gorlin-Gold cyst.
- Equal frequency in maxilla and mandible, most cases occur in incisor and canine region.
- No gender predilection.
- Peak incidence seen in second decade.
- COC is sometimes associated with odontogenic hamartomas or benign neoplasms.

Radiographically

Usually shows unilocular but a few have been multilocular radiolucency. Irregular calcified bodies of varying size and opacity may be seen in the radiolucent area.

Histopathological Picture

Histopathologically, COC consist of:

- The cyst lining shows proliferation to the point resembling ameloblastoma (i.e. basal columnar cells and suprabasal stellate and spindled cells in an arrangement that suggest stellate reticulum).
- Within this proliferation of epithelium, cells undergoing the characteristic 'ghost cell' keratinization is seen.
- Dystrophic calcification of the ghost cells may be seen.
- Dysplastic dentine may be laid down adjacent to the basal layer of the epithelium.

Additional Points

- Ghost cell keratinization may be observed in odontomas, ameloblastomas, ameloblastic fibro-odontomas, and in odontoameloblastoma.
- Different theories have been put forth to explain the pathogenesis of ghost cells, viz. local hypoxia and degeneration, form of coagulative necrosis, metaplastic transformation, abortive formation of enamel matrix, aberrant keratinization and/or accumulation of hardkeratin.
- Put in cyst category in WHO 2017 classification.

Odontogenic Tumors

Odontogenic tumors are unique to oral cavity and do not occur elsewhere in the body. These tumors are named so because of their origin from the odontogenic (tooth forming) apparatus.

Odontogenic tumors portray a variety of lesions ranging from hamartomatous tissue proliferation to neoplasms with benign or malignant behavior. Due to the wide range of biological behavior, controversies exist regarding their pathogenesis, classification and histopathological features.

WHO 2017 Classification

Odontogenic Carcinomas

- Ameloblastic carcinoma
- Primary intraosseous carcinoma
- Sclerosing odontogenic carcinoma
- Clear cell odontogenic carcinoma
- Ghost cell odontogenic carcinoma
- Odontogenic carcinosarcoma
- Odontogenic sarcomas.

Benign Epithelial Odontogenic Tumors

- Ameloblastoma
- Ameloblastoma, unicystic type
- Ameloblastoma, extraosseous/peripheral type
- Metastasizing ameloblastoma
- Squamous odontogenic tumor
- Calcifying epithelial odontogenic tumor
- Adenomatoid odontogenic tumor

Benign Mixed Epithelial and Mesenchymal Odontogenic Tumors

- Ameloblastic fibroma
- Primordial odontogenic tumor
- Odontoma
- Dentinogenic ghost cell tumor

Benign Mesenchymal Odontogenic Tumors

- Odontogenic fibroma
- Odontogenic myxoma/myxofibroma
- Cementoblastoma
- Cemento-ossifying fibroma.

UNICYSTIC AMELOBLASTOMA

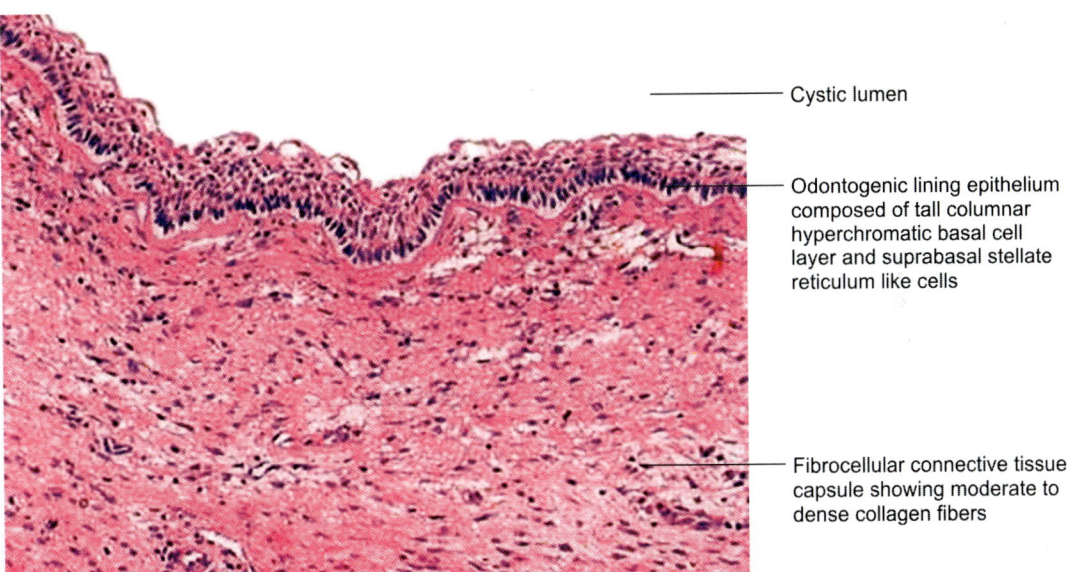

Cystic lumen

Odontogenic lining epithelium composed of tall columnar hyperchromatic basal cell layer and suprabasal stellate reticulum like cells

Fibrocellular connective tissue capsule showing moderate to dense collagen fibers

Fig. 2.1: 10X

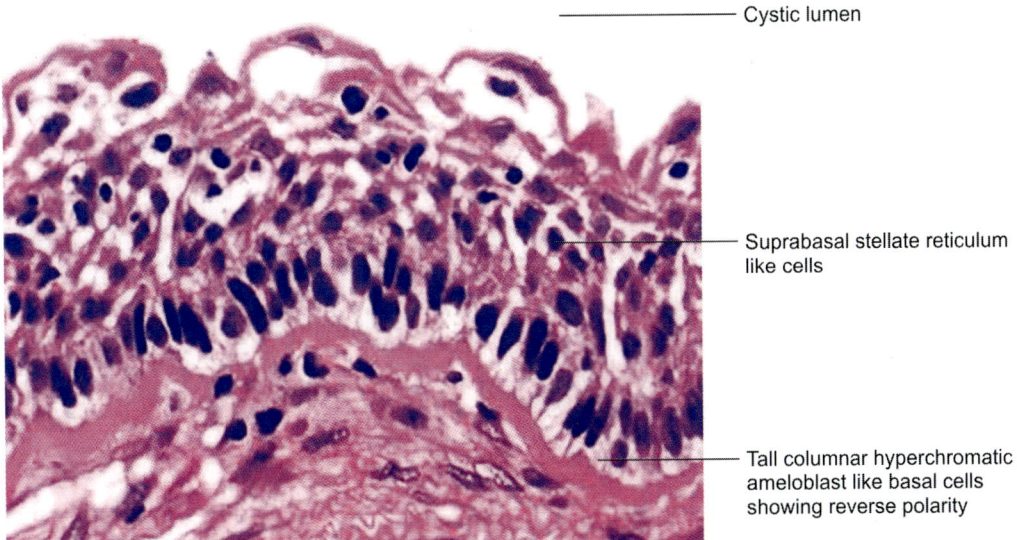

Cystic lumen

Suprabasal stellate reticulum like cells

Tall columnar hyperchromatic ameloblast like basal cells showing reverse polarity

Fig. 2.2: 40X

Key Points

- Unicystic ameloblastoma is the cystic variant of ameloblastoma an odontogenic tumor.
- Marked predominance for the posterior mandible, including the ascending ramus (molar—ramus region).
- Occurs in a younger population (average age 22.1 years) compared with conventional ameloblastomas.
- Male predominance with a male : female ratio of 1.6 : 1.
- Most of these lesions are associated with an impacted tooth, and the most commonly cited provisional diagnosis is dentigerous cyst.
- Radiographic appearance—unilocular and multilocular.

Histopathological Picture

- Microscopically, it shows cystic lumen lined by odontogenic lining epithelium with hyperchromatic tall columnar basal cell layer showing reverse polarity (ameloblast-like cell).
- Suprabasal cells resemble stellate reticulum.
- Basal cell show reverse polarity of the nuclei and a subnuclear vacuole is usually noted between the basement membrane and nucleus.
- Lining epithelium similar to those described by Vickers and Gorlin.

Histologic UA Subgrouping (Modified After Ackermann, et al.)

Subgroup Interpretation

1 Luminal UA
1.2 Luminal and intraluminal UA
1.2.3 Luminal, intraluminal, and intramural UA
1.3 Luminal and intramural UA

The luminal type is defined as having an odontogenic epithelial lining.

UA subgroup 1.2 shows simple luminal and intraluminal proliferation. UA subgroup 1.2.3 covers cases where there is an occurrence of luminal, intraluminal and intramural (wall) ameloblastoma.

The last subgroup (1.3) exhibits a cyst with a luminal lining in combination with intramural nodules of solid multicystic ameloblastoma (SMA) tissue.

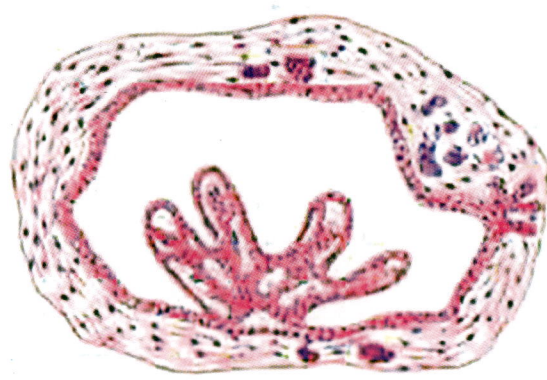

Fig. 2.3

SOLID/MULTICYSTIC AMELOBLASTOMA (SMA)

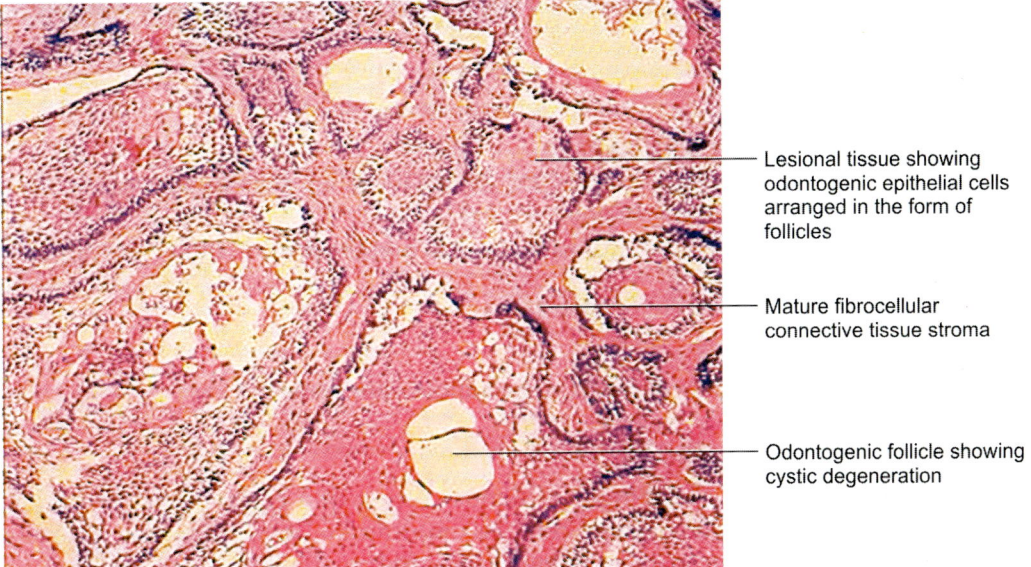

Lesional tissue showing odontogenic epithelial cells arranged in the form of follicles

Mature fibrocellular connective tissue stroma

Odontogenic follicle showing cystic degeneration

Fig. 2.4: 4X

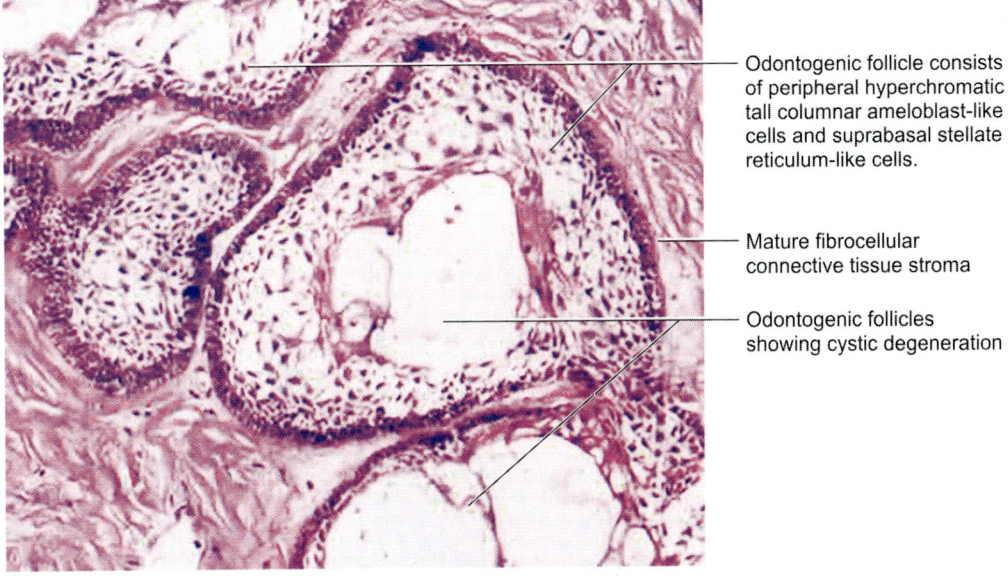

Odontogenic follicle consists of peripheral hyperchromatic tall columnar ameloblast-like cells and suprabasal stellate reticulum-like cells.

Mature fibrocellular connective tissue stroma

Odontogenic follicles showing cystic degeneration

Fig. 2.5: 10X

Key Points

- Benign odontogenic epithelial neoplasm.
- It is slow-growing but locally aggressive, with a high rate of recurrence, if not removed adequately.
- Average age of diagnosis is between 33 and 39 years.
- Mandibular molar-ramus area is most common site involved.
- Males are more affected then females.
- Tumors that continue to enlarge may cause the surrounding bone to become so thin that crepitation or eggshell crackling may be elicited.
- The typical picture (gross) is of a multilocular destruction of bone, but unilocular appearances also occur.

Radiographically

Unilocular or multilocular honeycomb or soap-bubble appearance.

Histopathological Picture

- Follicular ameloblastoma: Odontogenic islands consist of a central mass of polyhedral cells, or loosely connected angular cells resembling stellate reticulum, surrounded by a layer of cuboidal or columnar cells resembling inner enamel epithelium or preameloblast.
- Cystic degeneration commonly occurs within the follicles.
- Mature fibrous connective tissue stroma of moderate amount is seen.

Acanthomatous Ameloblastoma

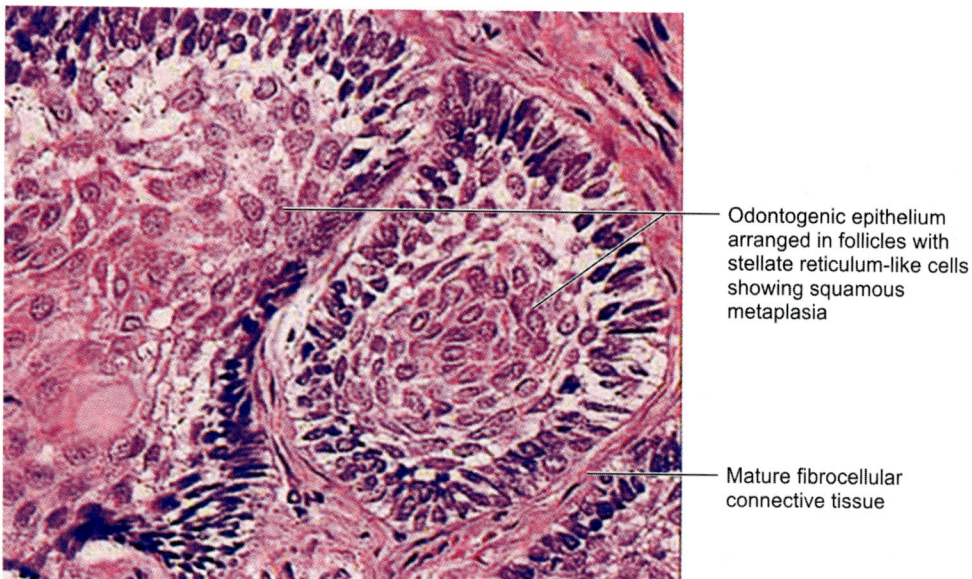

Odontogenic epithelium arranged in follicles with stellate reticulum-like cells showing squamous metaplasia

Mature fibrocellular connective tissue

Fig. 2.6: 40X

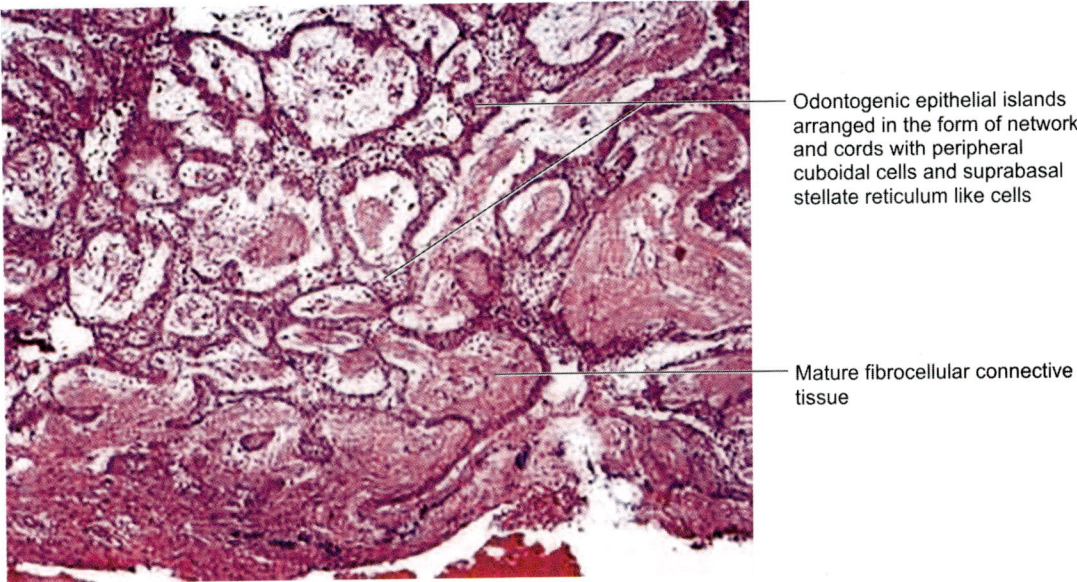

Odontogenic epithelial islands arranged in the form of network and cords with peripheral cuboidal cells and suprabasal stellate reticulum like cells

Mature fibrocellular connective tissue

Fig. 2.7: 4X

Histopathological Picture

- This term is applied when suprabasal stellate reticulum like cells show extensive squamous metaplasia.
- Sometimes keratin formation may be seen in the center of islands of tumor cells.
- The horny pearls may become calcified.
- Usually, the general pattern of this tumor is of the follicular type with squamous metaplasia.

Plexiform Ameloblastoma

- In the plexiform pattern tumor epithelium is arranged as a network which is bound by a layer of cuboidal to columnar cells and includes cells resembling stellate reticulum.
- Cystic degeneration occurs but is usually due to stromal degeneration rather than due to a cystic change within the epithelium.
- The supporting connective tissue stroma is loosely arranged and vascular.

DESMOPLASTIC AMELOBLASTOMA (DA)

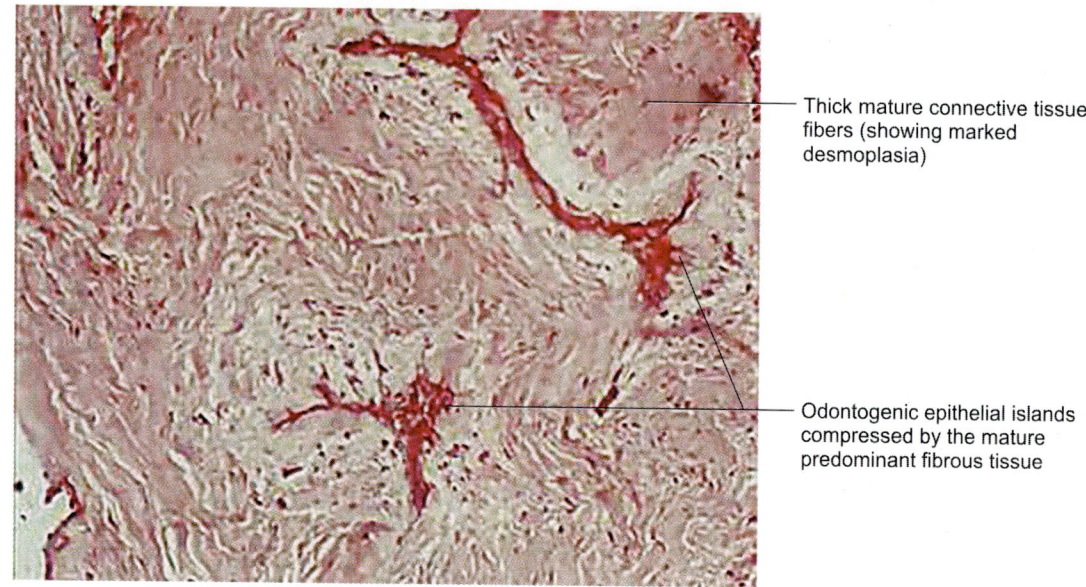

Thick mature connective tissue fibers (showing marked desmoplasia)

Odontogenic epithelial islands compressed by the mature predominant fibrous tissue

Fig. 2.8: 10X

Key Points

- Desmoplastic ameloblastoma (DA) is a benign, locally infiltrative epithelial neoplasm believed to be a variant or subtype of the SMA.
- Equal distribution in location between the maxilla and mandible.
- DA occurs in the age range from 17 to 83 years with a mean age of 41.9 years.
- Predilection for premolar-molar region
- The radiographic features of DA varies from unilocular radiolucent to multilocular or mixed radiolucent/radiopaque in 53% of the cases.
- Mixed radiolucent and radio-opaque appearance may be confused with fibro-osseous lesion.
- This term is used, especially in the follicular type of tumor, when there is a marked hyalinization (desmoplasia) of the connective tissue stroma.

Histopathological Picture

- Tumor islands in desmoplastic ameloblastoma are often very irregular in shape with a pointed stellate appearance. The morphology of these islands is often bizarre with an almost pathognomonic 'animal-like (kite-like)' configuration or outline.
- The epithelial cells at the periphery of the islands are cuboidal. Occasionally with hyperchromatic nuclei. Columnar cells demonstrating reversed nuclear polarity are rarely conspicuous, although an occasional isolated island may exhibit focal ameloblasts like peripheral cells.
- Abundant thick collagen fibers that seem to compress or 'squeeze' the odontogenic epithelial islands from the periphery.
- Formation of metaplastic bone trabeculae (osteoplasia) rimmed by active osteoblasts has been described in several cases.

ADENOMATOID ODONTOGENIC TUMOR (AOT)

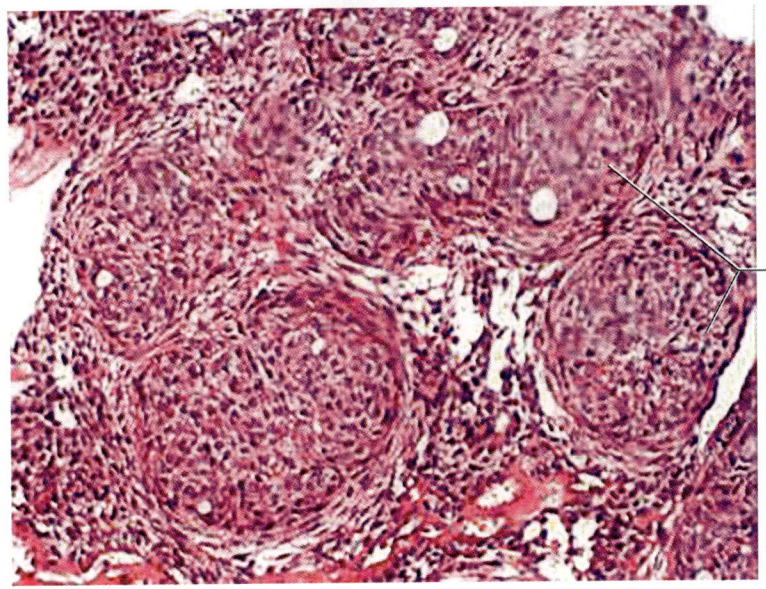

Odontogenic epithelial cells arranged in nodular and rosette pattern

Fig. 2.9: 10X

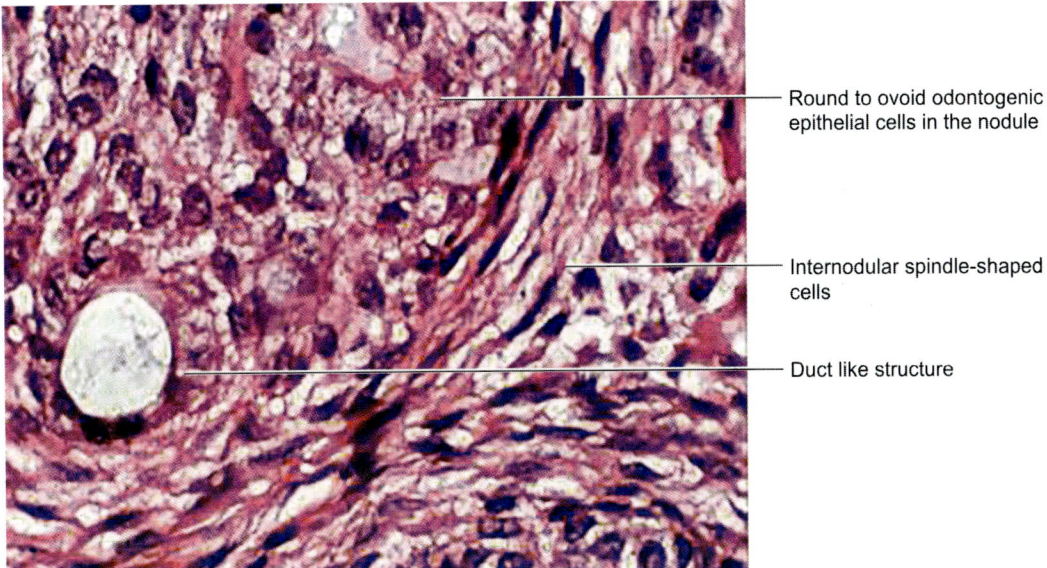

Round to ovoid odontogenic epithelial cells in the nodule

Internodular spindle-shaped cells

Duct like structure

Fig. 2.10: 40X

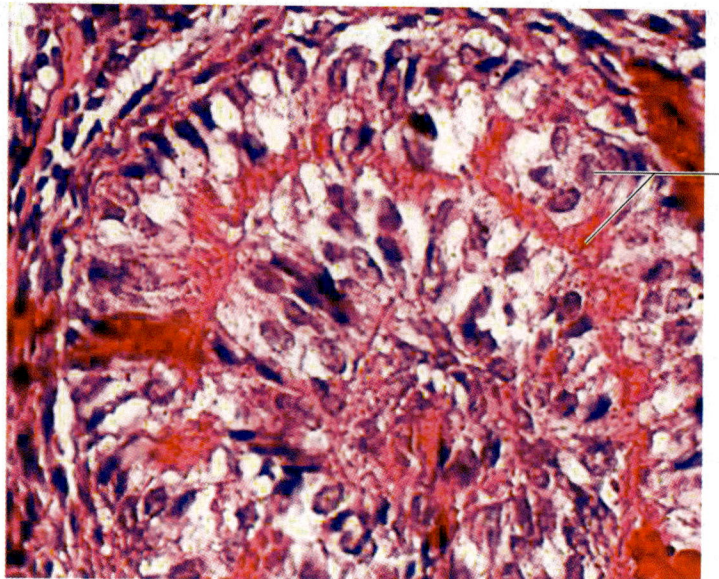

Double convoluted pattern with eosinophilic material

Fig. 2.11: 40X

Key Points
- Also known as 2/3rd tumor because 2/3rd cases
  a. Occurs in females.
  b. Present in maxillary anterior region.
  c. Associated with impacted canine.
- Initially, it was thought to be mixed odontogenic tumor now, it is considered as pure epithelial odontogenic tumor.
- Controversy exists whether it is a cyst, tumor or hamartoma.
- Age distribution 3 to 82 years of age, its predilection for young patients is well-established.

Histopathological Picture
- The AOT exhibits diverse histomorphologic features but the light microscopic findings are remarkably consistent.
- AOT is made-up of a cellular multinodular proliferation of spindle, cuboidal, and columnar cells in a variety of patterns; usually scattered, duct like structures, eosinophilic material, and calcifications in several forms, and a fibrous capsule of variable thickness.
- Droplets of eosinophilic material are seen in between the spindle and polygonal cells (hyaline droplet).
- The duct like or microcyst lumina frequently are lined by an eosinophilic rim of varying thickness the so-called 'hyaline ring'.

CALCIFYING EPITHELIAL ODONTOGENIC TUMOR/(CEOT)

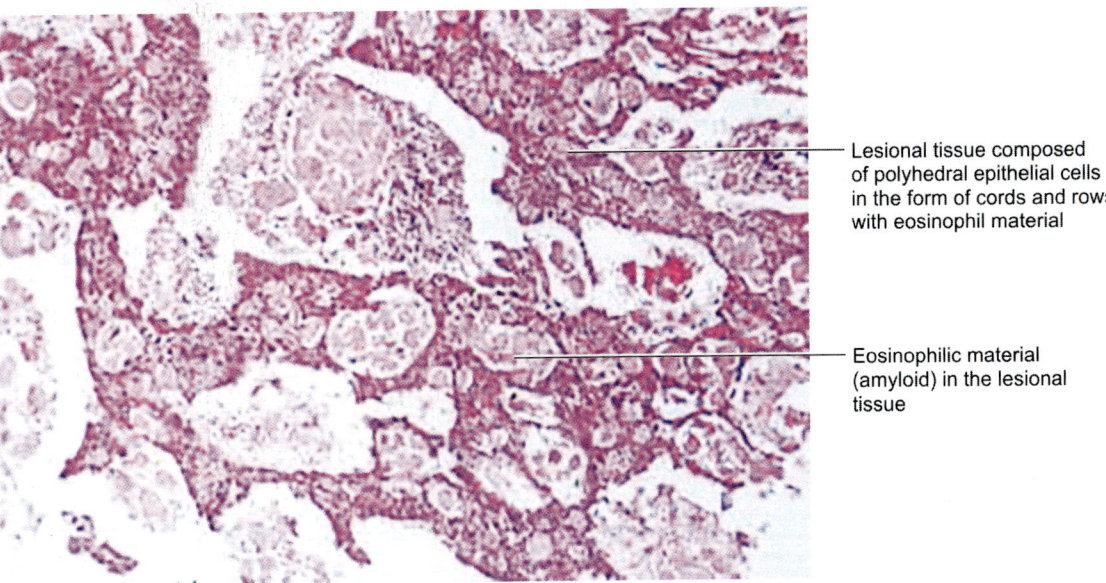

Lesional tissue composed of polyhedral epithelial cells in the form of cords and rows with eosinophil material

Eosinophilic material (amyloid) in the lesional tissue

Fig. 2.12: 4X (*Courtesy:* Department of Oral Pathology, GDCH, Aurangabad)

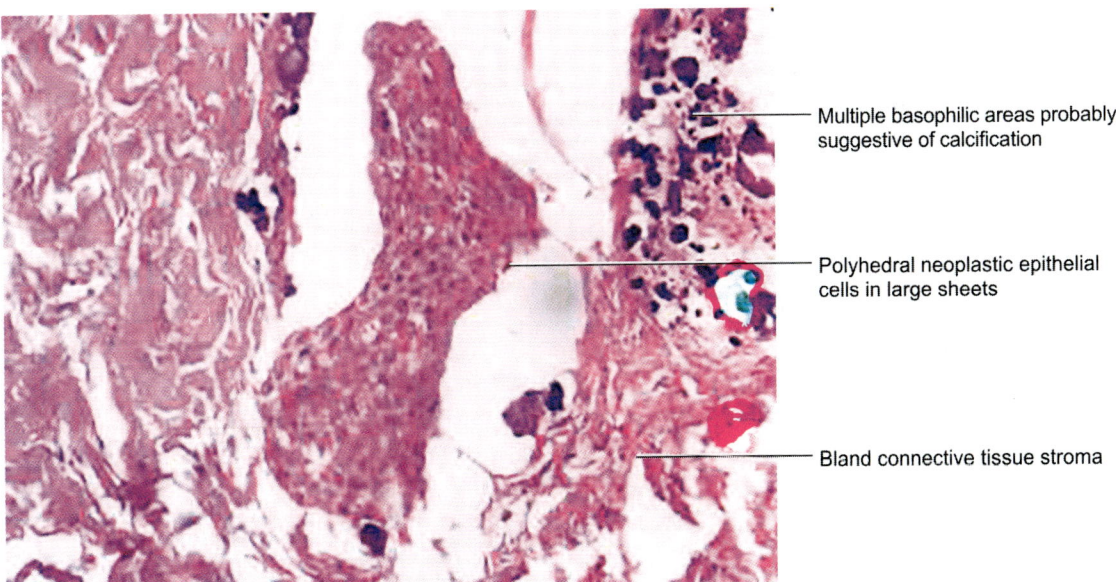

Multiple basophilic areas probably suggestive of calcification

Polyhedral neoplastic epithelial cells in large sheets

Bland connective tissue stroma

Fig. 2.13: 4X (*Courtesy:* Department of Oral Pathology, GDCH, Aurangabad)

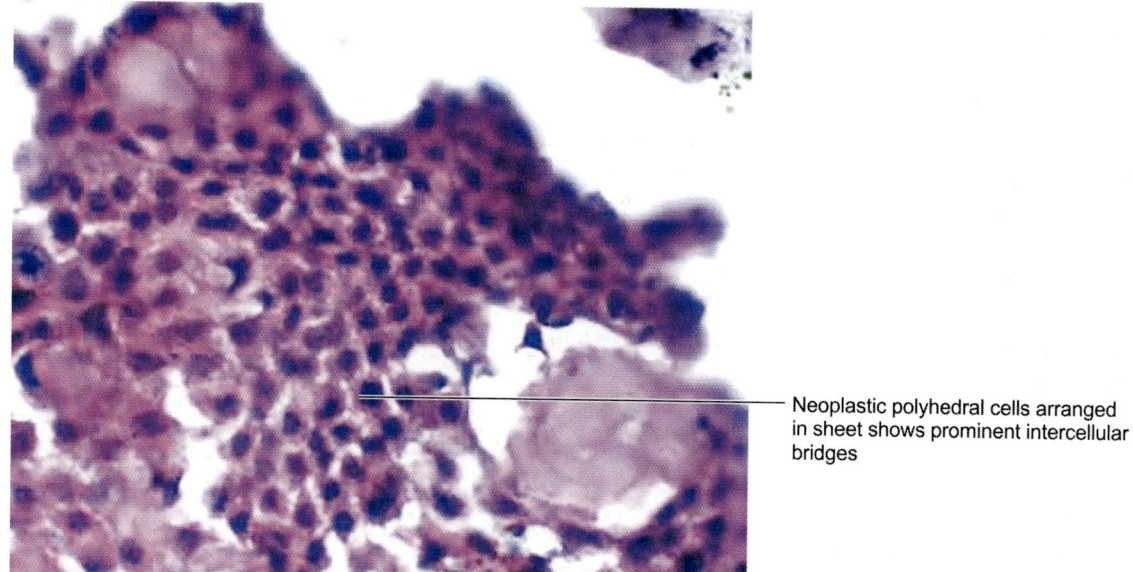

Neoplastic polyhedral cells arranged in sheet shows prominent intercellular bridges

Fig. 2.14: 40X (*Courtesy:* Department of Oral Pathology, GDCH, Aurangabad)

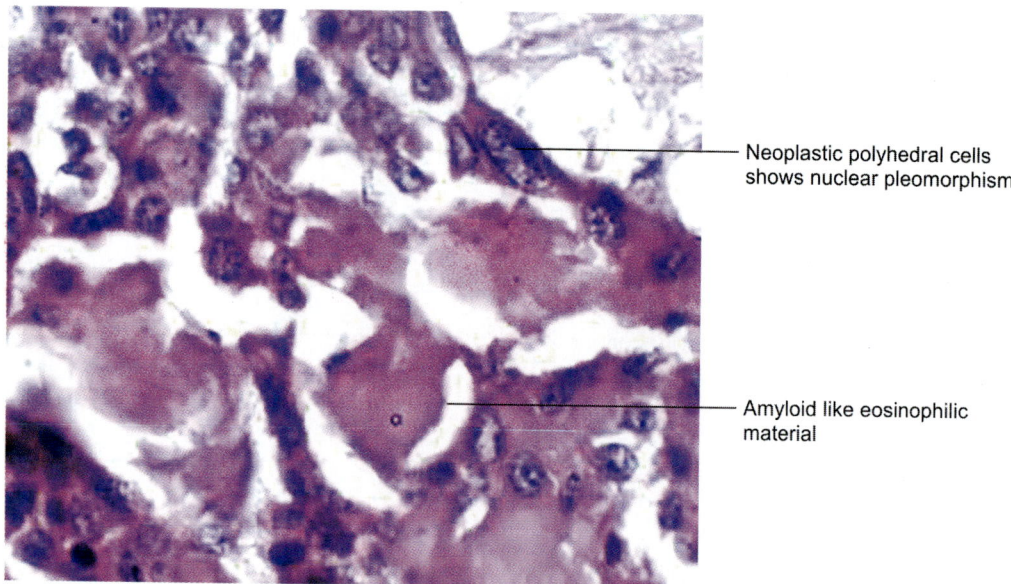

Neoplastic polyhedral cells shows nuclear pleomorphism

Amyloid like eosinophilic material

Fig. 2.15: 40X (*Courtesy:* Department of Oral Pathology, GDCH, Aurangabad)

Key Points

- Other name is Pindborg tumor.
- First described Dr Jens J Pindborg in 1956.
- Thought to arise from stratum intermedium or remnants of the primitive dental lamina.
- Mean age is 40 years at time of diagnosis in both men and women, with a range of 8–92 years.
- Predilection for mandible, 2 : 1 (molar region).

Radiographically

Tumor contains foci of calcification. These scattered flecks of calcification throughout the radiolucency give 'driven snow' appearance.

Histopathological Picture

- Histologically CEOT is composed of polyhedral epithelial cells with prominent intracellular bridges.
- These polyhedral cells are closely packed in large sheets, sometimes show cord and island.
- Nuclear pleomorphism is frequently noted.
- Connective tissue stroma bland and fibrous.
- Homogeneous, eosinophilic substance which is interpreted as amyloid, glycoprotein, basal lamina, keratin or enamel matrix is also seen (characteristic microscopic features).
- Calcifications is also seen either as dystrophic type or in the form of Liesegang rings.

Additional Point

Clear cell component can be seen in CEOT which is called clear cell variant of CEOT.

MYXOMA

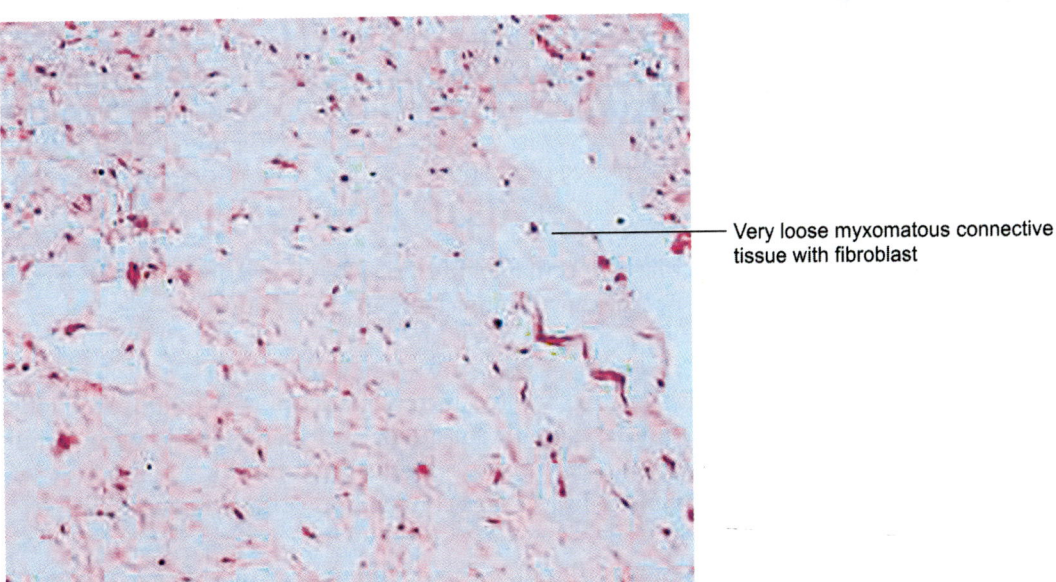

Very loose myxomatous connective tissue with fibroblast

Fig. 2.16: 10X

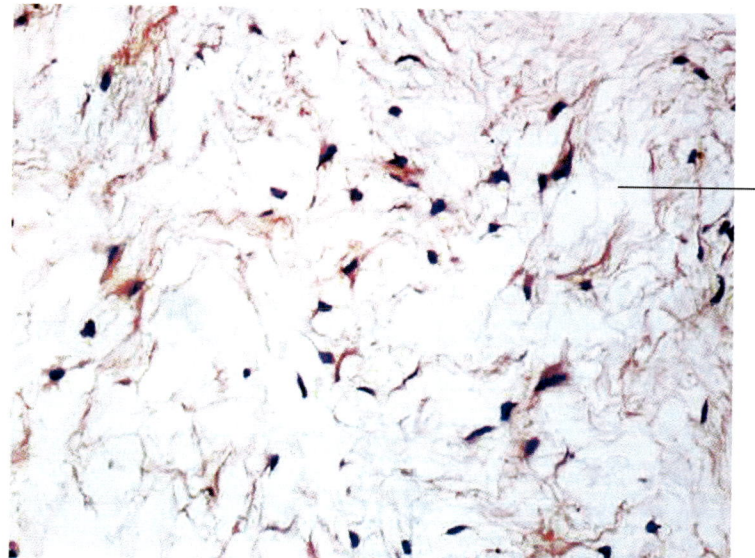

Loose basophilic myxomatous tissue with round to spindle-shaped fibroblast

Fig. 2.17: 40X

Key Points

- Locally aggressive neoplasm.
- Traditionally, the myxoma of the maxilla and mandible has been considered to be a neoplasm of odontogenic origin.
  Although the evidence is mainly circumstantial, support of an odontogenic origin has been perpetuated by:
  - a. It is almost exclusive occurrence in the tooth-bearing areas of the jaws.
  - b. Frequent occurrence in young individuals.
  - c. Common association with an unerupted tooth or a developmentally absent tooth.
  - d. Histologic resemblance to dental mesenchyme, especially the dental papilla.
  - e. The occasional presence of sparse amounts of odontogenic epithelium.
- The neoplasm's odontogenic derivation is believed to originate from the primitive mesenchymal portion of the developing tooth germ (dental follicle, dental papilla, and periodontal ligament) as an inductive effect of nests of odontogenic epithelium on mesenchymal tissue or as a direct myxomatous change of fibrous tissue in an odontogenic fibroma.
- Myxoma is common in the mandible, molar-premolar region.
- No sex predilection.
- Radiographically, the multilocular trabecular pattern has been described as 'honeycomb', 'soap bubble', 'tennis racket', 'wispy', and 'spider web' in appearance.

Histopathological Picture

- Histologically, the odontogenic myxoma is bland in appearance and is composed of loosely arranged, evenly dispersed spindle-shaped, rounded, and stellate cells with a lightly eosinophilic cytoplasm in a mucoid rich (myxoid), intercellular matrix.
- The myxoid matrix is rich in hyaluronic acid and chondroitin sulfate (hence stains more basophilic with H&E).
- Myxomas have a fine network of reticulin fibers, and some have low collagen content.
- Terms fibromyxoma and myxofibroma are used when myxomatous component is more or fibrous component is more respectively.

- An occasional island or rest of inactive-appearing odontogenic epithelium may be found.
- A dental follicle or odontogenic fibroma should be considered in differential diagnosis if myxomatous tissue contains islands or cords of odontogenic epithelium.
- Odontogenic myxomas lack the epithelial lining found in many dental follicles.

ODONTOME

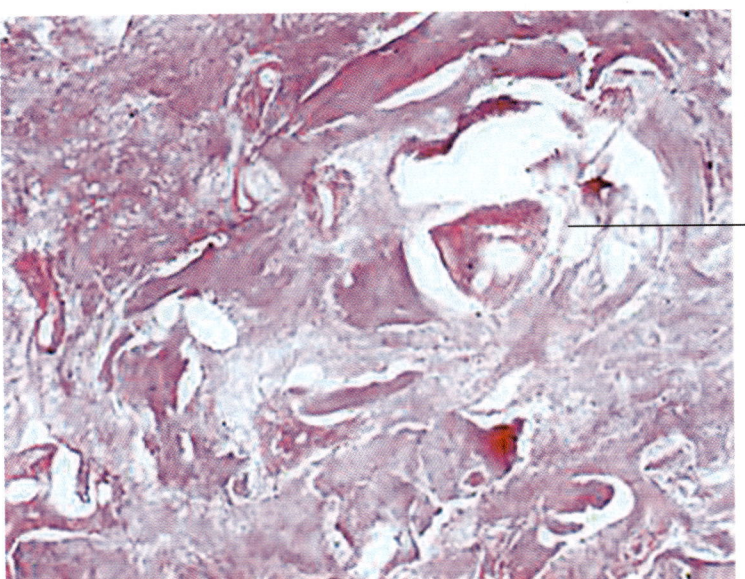

Decalcified section showing multiple hard tissue structure probably dentin and cementum like areas

Fig. 2.18: 4X

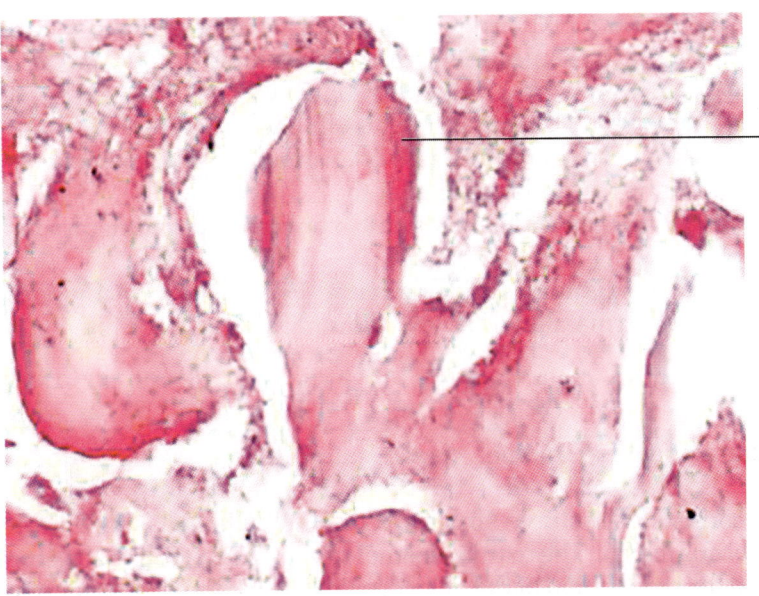

Dysplastic dentin admixed with irregular, curvilinear clefts suggestive of lost enamel during decalcification

Fig. 2.19: 10X

Compound Odontome

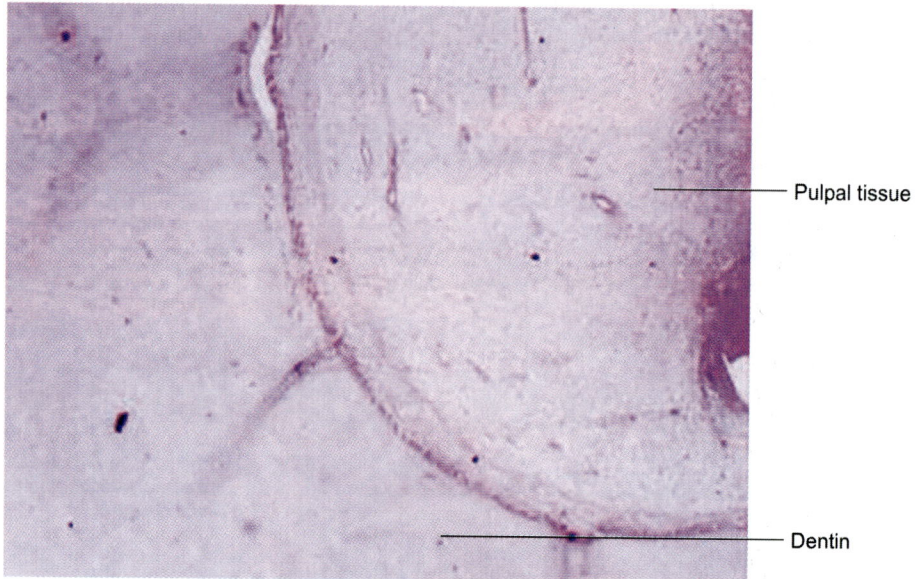

Fig. 2.20: 4X

Key Points

- In WHO classification classified under 'Tumors containing odontogenic epithelium with odontogenic ectomesenchyme, with or without dental hard tissue formation'.
- Some authors considered them as hamartomas rather than a true neoplasm.
- Two types—complex and compound odontome.
- The WHO defines complex odontoma as a malformation in which all of the dental tissues are represented, and individual tissues mainly are well-formed but occur in a disorderly pattern.
- The compound odontoma is defined as a malformation in which all of the dental tissues are represented in a more orderly pattern than in the complex odontoma so that the lesion consists of many tooth-like structures.
- The compound odontoma is composed of multiple small tooth like structures.
- The complex odontoma consists of a conglomerate mass of enamel, dentin, cementum and pulp tissue which bears no anatomic resemblance to a tooth.
- It is often difficult to differentiate clinically and histologically between supernumerary teeth and compound odontomas.
- Although compound and complex odontomas may be found in any site, the compound type is more often seen in the anterior maxilla; complex odontomas occur more often in the molar regions of either jaw.

Histopathological Picture

- Odontomas contain varying amounts of enamel, dentin, pulp tissue and cementum-like tissue.
- The compound odontoma consists of multiple structures resembling small, single rooted teeth, contained in a loose fibrous matrix. The mature enamel caps of the tooth-like structures are lost during decalcification for preparation of the microscopic section, but varying amounts of enamel matrix are often present.

- Pulp tissue often is seen in the normal location.
- Complex odontomas consist largely of mature tubular dentin. This dentin encloses clefts or hollow circular structures that contained the mature enamel which is removed during decalcification. The spaces may contain small amounts of enamel matrix or immature enamel.

Additional Points

- It is also considered as a type of supernumerary teeth.
- Ghost cells can also be seen in odontomas.

AMELOBLASTIC FIBROMA

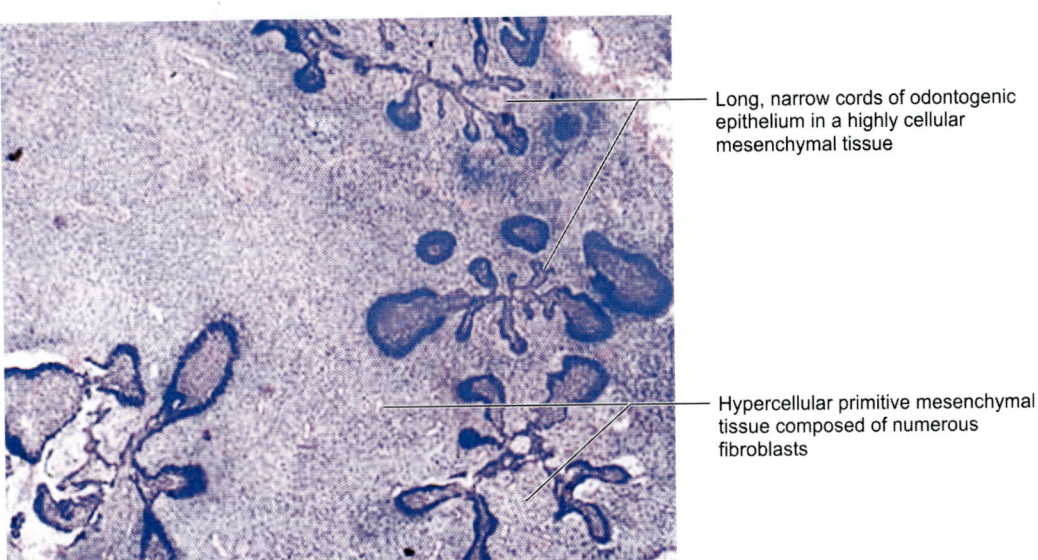

Long, narrow cords of odontogenic epithelium in a highly cellular mesenchymal tissue

Hypercellular primitive mesenchymal tissue composed of numerous fibroblasts

Fig. 2.21: 4X

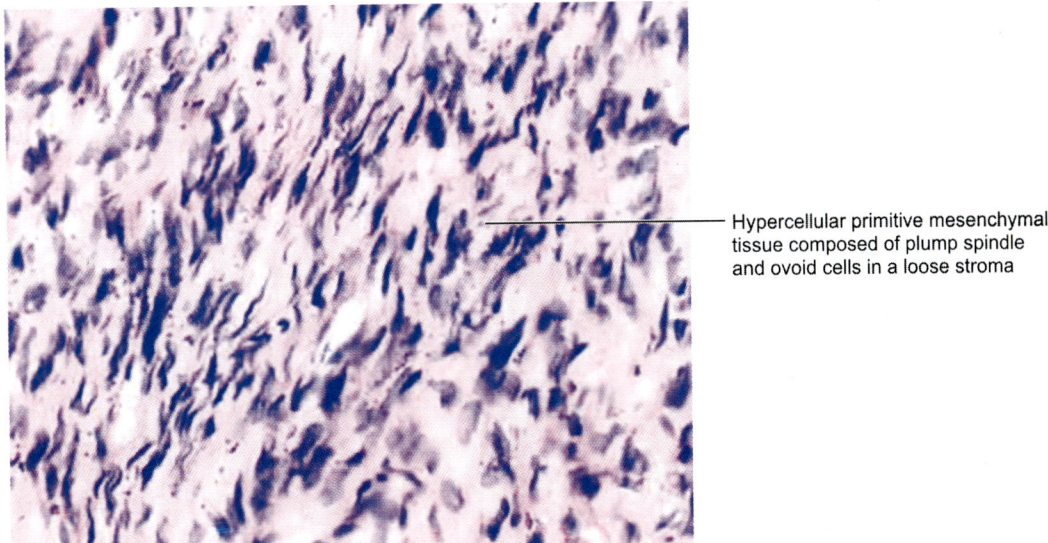

Hypercellular primitive mesenchymal tissue composed of plump spindle and ovoid cells in a loose stroma

Fig. 2.22: 10X

Key Points

- These neoplasms occur predominantly in children and young adults usually within an age range of 6 months to 42 years (average age, 14.6–15.5 years).
- The posterior mandible is the most common site, and about 80% of cases are located in the first permanent molar and second primary molar area.
- Slight male predilection.
- The neoplasm appears as a well-defined, unilocular or multilocular radiolucency with a smooth, well-defined outline and often with a sclerotic opaque border.

Histopathological Picture

- AF is a mixed tumor in which the epithelial and connective tissue components are neoplastic.
- The epithelial component is characterized by proliferating islands, cords, and strands of odontogenic epithelium exhibiting a peripheral layer of cuboidal or columnar cells, and the central area resembles the stellate reticulum of the embryonic enamel organ.
- The ectomesenchymal component is that of an embryonic, cell-rich mesenchyme that mimics the dental papilla.
- The cells are rounded or angular and are fibroblast-like, with little collagen. The degree of cellularity varies within the same tumor and between tumors.

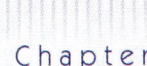

Reactive Lesions of the Oral Cavity

FIBROEPITHELIAL HYPERPLASIA

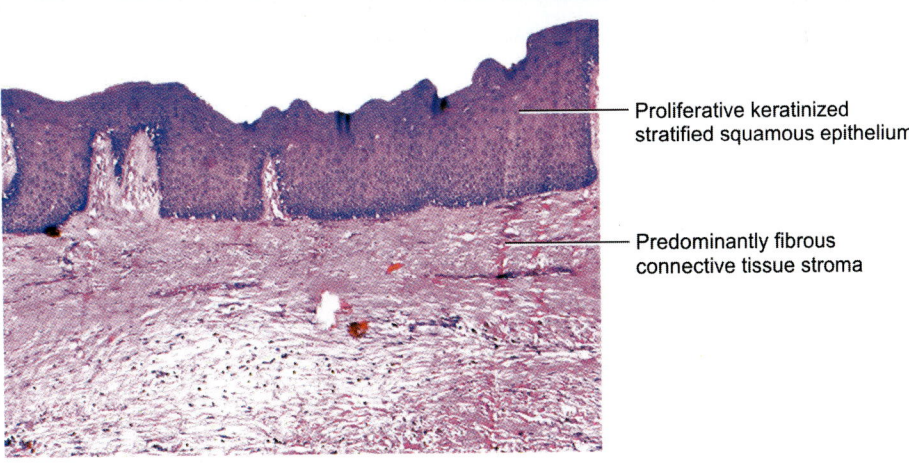

Proliferative keratinized stratified squamous epithelium

Predominantly fibrous connective tissue stroma

Fig. 3.1: 4X

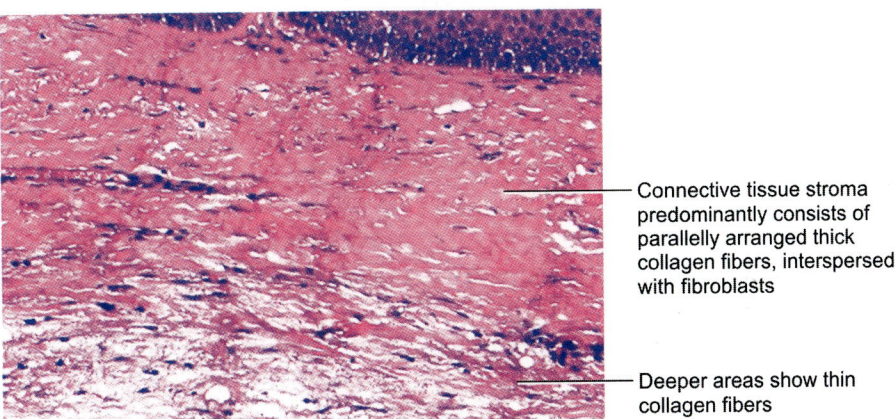

Connective tissue stroma predominantly consists of parallelly arranged thick collagen fibers, interspersed with fibroblasts

Deeper areas show thin collagen fibers

Fig. 3.2: 10X

Key Points

- Related to injury or chronic irritation (calculus, plaque), drugs, systemic conditions.
- Color also varies depending on cellularity, duration of lesion.
- Older lesions are pale pink in color.
- Surface is smooth or lobulated.

Histopathological Picture

- Proliferative parakeratinized stratified squamous epithelium.
- Basal cells appear to be hyperchromatic with elongated rete ridges.
- Fibrocellular connective tissue stroma, intense inflammatory cells.
- The connective tissue picture varies depending upon duration of the lesion.
- Usually fibrous component is more and cellular component is less in long-standing lesions.
- Reactive bone formation and dystropic calcification can also be seen.

IRRITATIONAL FIBROMA

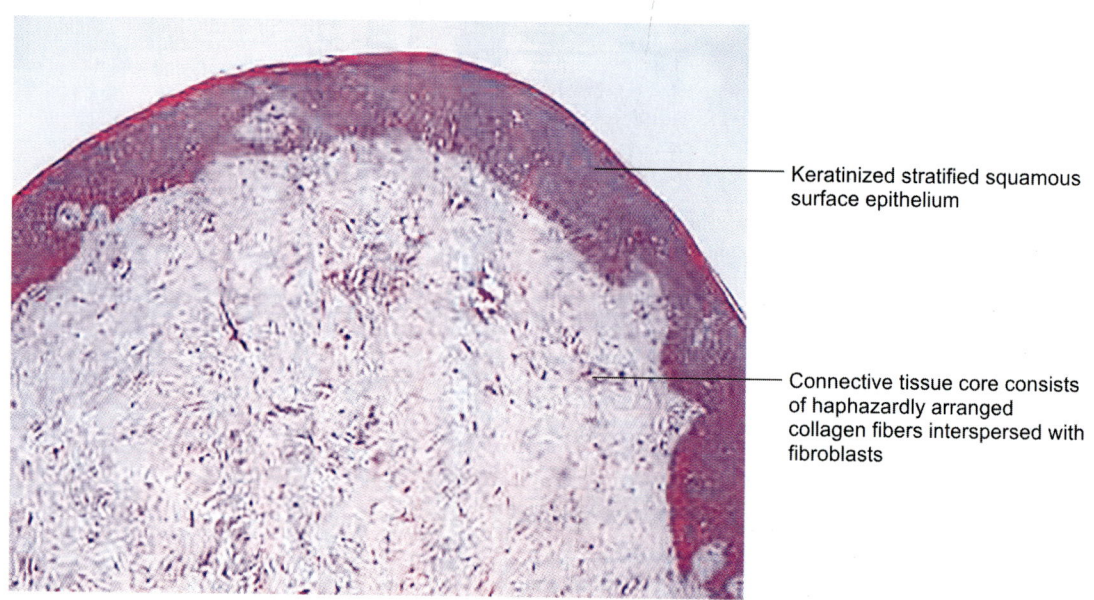

Keratinized stratified squamous surface epithelium

Connective tissue core consists of haphazardly arranged collagen fibers interspersed with fibroblasts

Fig. 3.3: 4X

Key Points

- Most common benign soft tissue neoplasm occurring in the oral cavity. However, some consider it as a reactive lesion.
- Commonly seen on buccal mucosa along the plane of occlusion. Other frequent sites are the gingiva, the tongue, lips and the palate.
- Can occur at any age but is most common in the third, fourth and fifth decade.

- Females are affected twice as frequently as males but some studies show predominance in male.
- Growth is nodular with smooth surface.
- Chronic cheek bite, trauma is the cause.

Histopathological Picture

- Fibrocellular connective tissue core covered by surface epithelium.
- Depending upon the cellularity (fibroblast) termed acellular/hypocellular or cellular/hypercellular fibroma.
- Collagen fibers are arranged haphazardly or in whorled pattern and interspersed with varying number of fibroblasts.
- The surface of the lesion is covered by a layer of stratified squamous epithelium which frequently appears stretched and shows shortening and flattening of the rete pegs (older lesions).
- If trauma to the tissue has occurred, vasodilatation, edema and inflammatory cell infiltration and superficial ulceration may be present.
- Areas of diffuse or focal calcification or even ossification are found in some fibromas.

PERIPHERAL CEMENTO-OSSIFYING FIBROMA

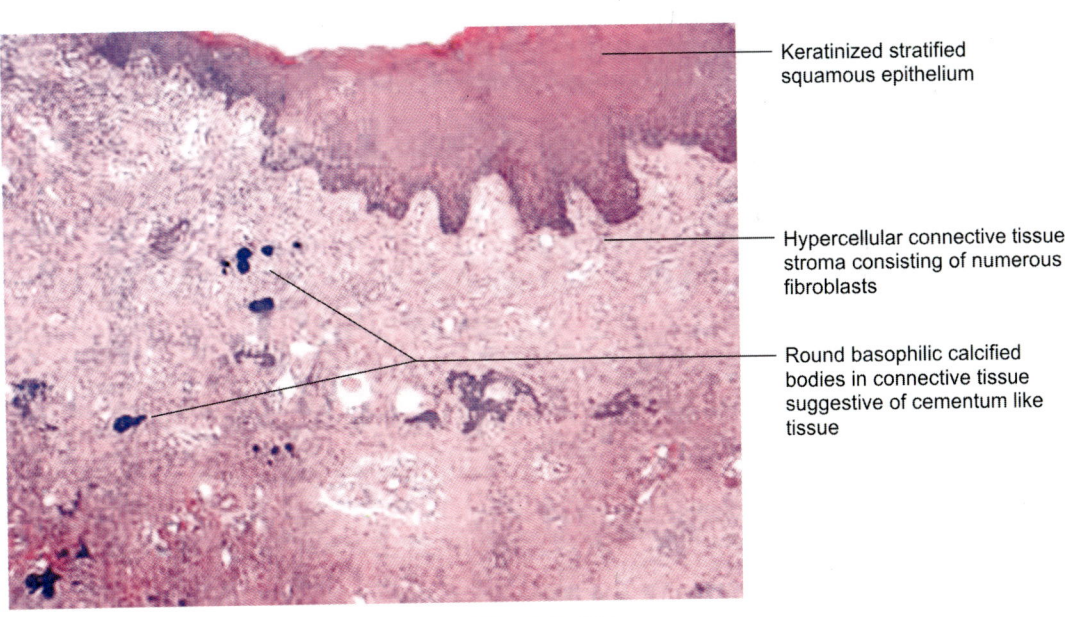

Keratinized stratified squamous epithelium

Hypercellular connective tissue stroma consisting of numerous fibroblasts

Round basophilic calcified bodies in connective tissue suggestive of cementum like tissue

Fig. 3.4: 4X

Key Points

- The term peripheral cemento-ossifying fibroma will be used here for that relatively common gingival lesion characterized by a high degree of cellularity usually exhibiting bone formation, although occasionally cementum-like material or rarely dystrophic calcification may be found instead.

- It is not considered to be the extraosseous counterpart of the central ossifying fibroma (which is a tumor and not peripheral one).
- Some investigators believe it to be originating from periodontal ligament.
- Female predilection 2 : 1 to 3 : 2.
- Lesions are approximately equally divided between the maxilla and the mandible.
- Clinically, it is a well-demarcated focal mass of tissue on the gingiva, with a sessile or pedunculated base.
- Color may resemble normal mucosa or slightly reddened. The surface may be intact or ulcerated.

Histopathological Picture

- Predominantly lesional tissue is comprised of large numbers of plump proliferating fibroblasts intermingled throughout a very delicate fibrillar stroma.
- Several forms of calcification can be seen.
- These calcification may be in the form of single or multiple interconnecting trabeculae of bone or osteoid (either mature lamellar bone or immature (woven) cellular bone).
- Sometime basophilic globular calcified areas resembling cementum are also seen.
- Dystrophic calcification may be noted.

PYOGENIC GRANULOMA

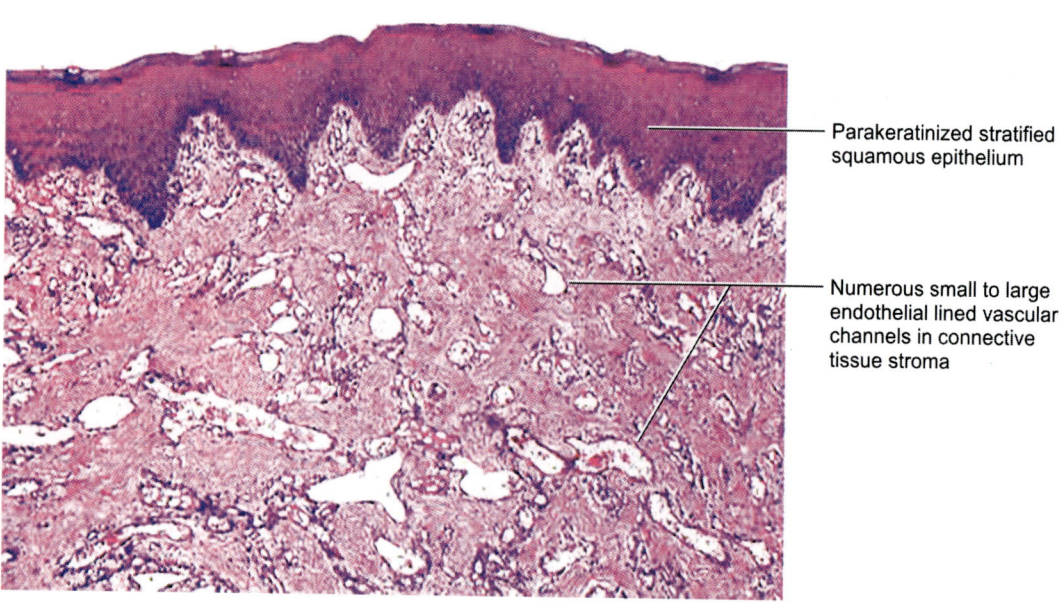

Parakeratinized stratified squamous epithelium

Numerous small to large endothelial lined vascular channels in connective tissue stroma

Fig. 3.5: 4X

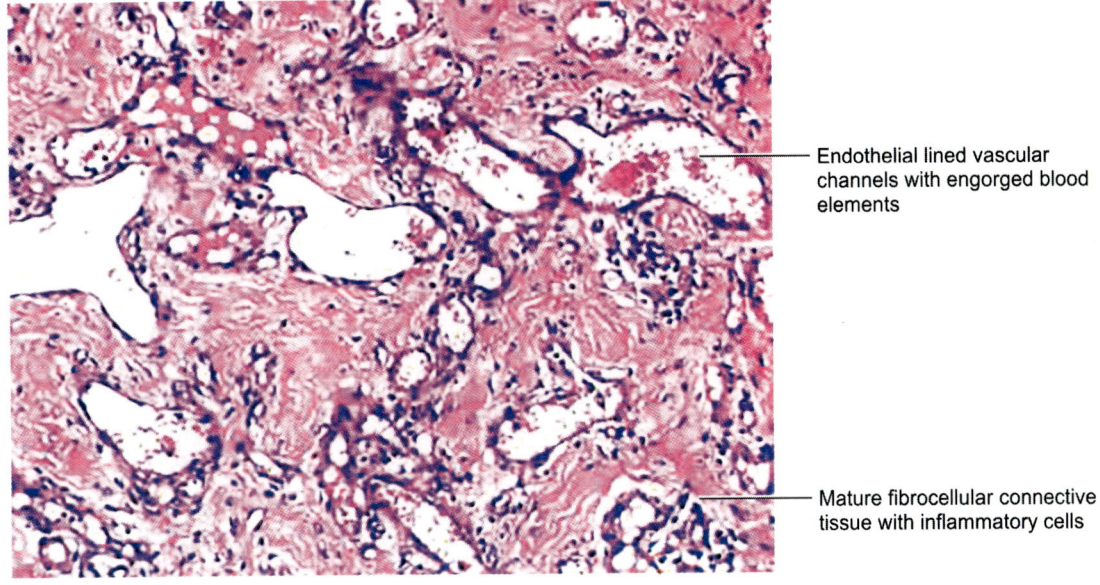

Endothelial lined vascular channels with engorged blood elements

Mature fibrocellular connective tissue with inflammatory cells

Fig. 3.6: 10X

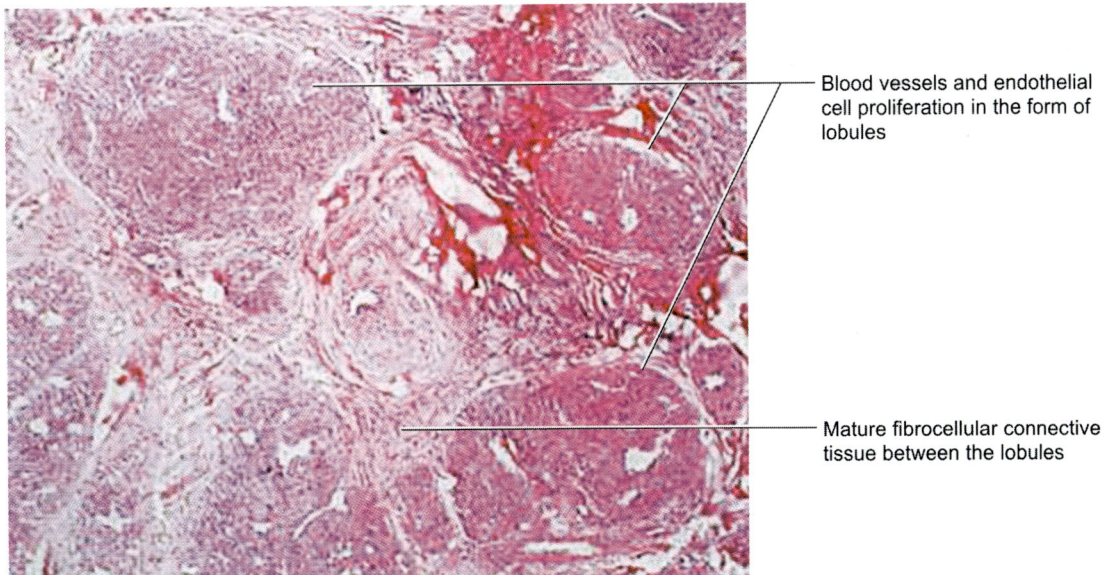

Blood vessels and endothelial cell proliferation in the form of lobules

Mature fibrocellular connective tissue between the lobules

Fig. 3.7: 4X

Key Points

- Term pyogenic granuloma is a misnomer as it was originally thought to be caused by pyogenic organisms but is now believed to be unrelated to infection.
- Histologically, it resembles angiomatous lesion rather than granulomatous lesion indicating that the term 'pyogenic granuloma' itself is a misnomer.
- Pyogenic granuloma arises as a result of some minor trauma to the tissues, which provides a pathway for the invasion of nonspecific types of microorganisms.
- The tissues respond in a characteristic manner to these organisms of low virulence by the overzealous proliferation of vascular type connective tissue.
- The surface of the pyogenic granuloma, especially in areas of ulceration, abounds with typical colonies of saprophytic microorganisms.
- Females are more affected because of hormonal effects on the vascular structures.
- Around 75% of all cases occur in gingiva, other sites involved are lips, tongue and buccal mucosa.
- It occurs more common on the facial aspect than the lingual or palatal aspects of gingiva.
- The lesion is more common in the maxillary anterior region than the posterior region.
- It usually presents as an elevated, pedunculated or sessile vascular mass with a smooth, lobulated surface, which commonly is ulcerated and shows a tendency for hemorrhage either spontaneously or upon slight trauma.
- It is deep red or reddish purple in color, depending upon its vascularity, often painless and rather soft in consistency.

Histopathological Picture

- The overlying epithelium, if present, is generally thin and atrophic, but may be hyperplastic.
- Ulcerated lesions shows a fibrinous exudate of varying thickness over its surface.
- Presence of numerous endothelium-lined vascular spaces and budding endothelial cells along with the proliferation of fibroblasts.
- Both clinically and microscopically, an old lesion may resemble a fibroepithelial polyp or even a typical fibroma, and it is likely that many so-called intraoral fibromas are healed pyogenic granulomas.
- Pregnancy tumor is histologically identical to pyogenic granuloma of the gingiva frequently occurring during pregnancy and often has been called the pregnancy tumor.

Additional Point

Pyogenic granuloma is also called 'lobular capillary hemangioma'.

PERIPHERAL GIANT CELL GRANULOMA (PGCG)

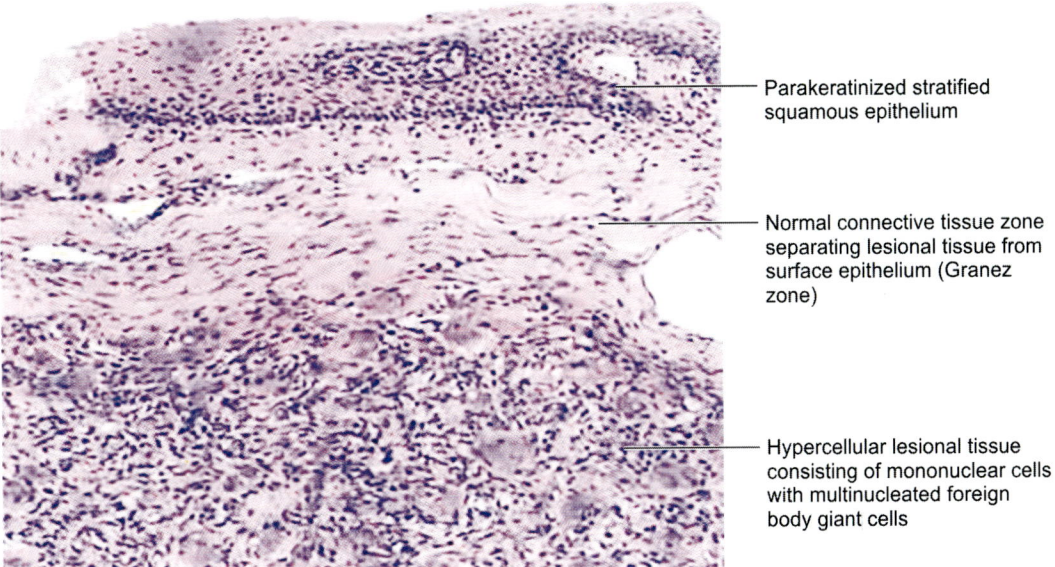

Parakeratinized stratified squamous epithelium

Normal connective tissue zone separating lesional tissue from surface epithelium (Granez zone)

Hypercellular lesional tissue consisting of mononuclear cells with multinucleated foreign body giant cells

Fig. 3.8: 4X

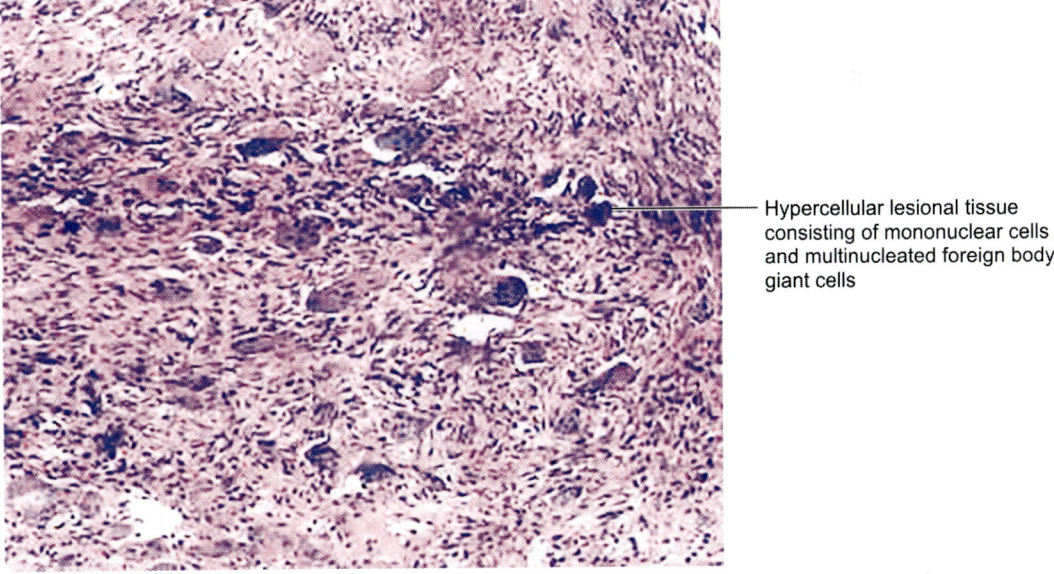

Hypercellular lesional tissue consisting of mononuclear cells and multinucleated foreign body giant cells

Fig. 3.9: 40X

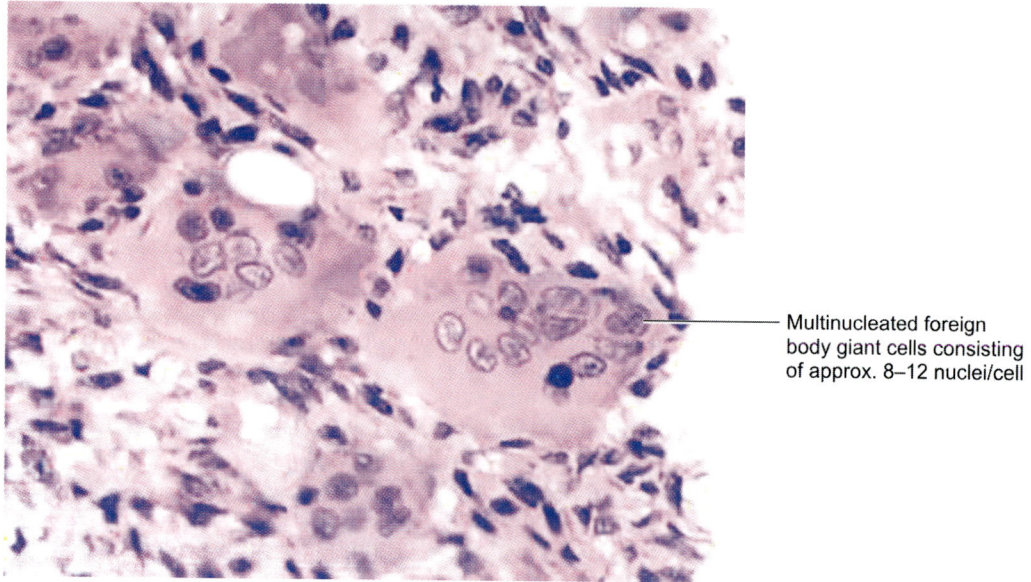

Multinucleated foreign body giant cells consisting of approx. 8–12 nuclei/cell

Fig. 3.10: 40X

Key Points

- Relatively frequent, non-neoplastic, tumor-like reactive lesion occurring exclusively on gingiva/alveolar crest.
- Thought to arise from the periodontal ligament or the periosteum following local irritation or chronic trauma.
- Clinically, it may bear resemblance to pyogenic granuloma and peripheral ossifying fibroma.
- PGCG occurs most frequently anterior to the molars with slight female predilection.
- PGCG manifests as a red-purple nodule located on gingiva or edentulous alveolar margins, fundamentally in the lower jaw.
- The lesion can develop at any age, though it is more common between the fifth and sixth decade of life.
- The color may range from dark red to reddish blue and the surface is occasionally ulcerated.
- Consistency of lesion varies from soft to rubbery to firm.

Histopathological Picture

- Lesional tissue composed of abundant ovoid, spindle or fusiform mononuclear-shaped cells and multinucleated giant cells.
- A zone of dense connective tissue (pseudocapsule) separating the giant cell proliferation from superficial epithelial surface is seen and termed 'Grenz zone'.
- Newly formed lesions are frequently cellular and contain plump to ovoid fibroblast while mature lesions show more of spindle-shaped cells.
- The lesions typically contains abundant capillaries. Hemorrhagic foci are also typical, with the release of hemosiderin pigment and invasion by mononuclear phagocytes and inflammatory cells.
- Osteoid tissue and bone formation is not an unusual finding in PGCG.

Giant Cell Lesions

CENTRAL GIANT CELL GRANULOMA (CGCG)

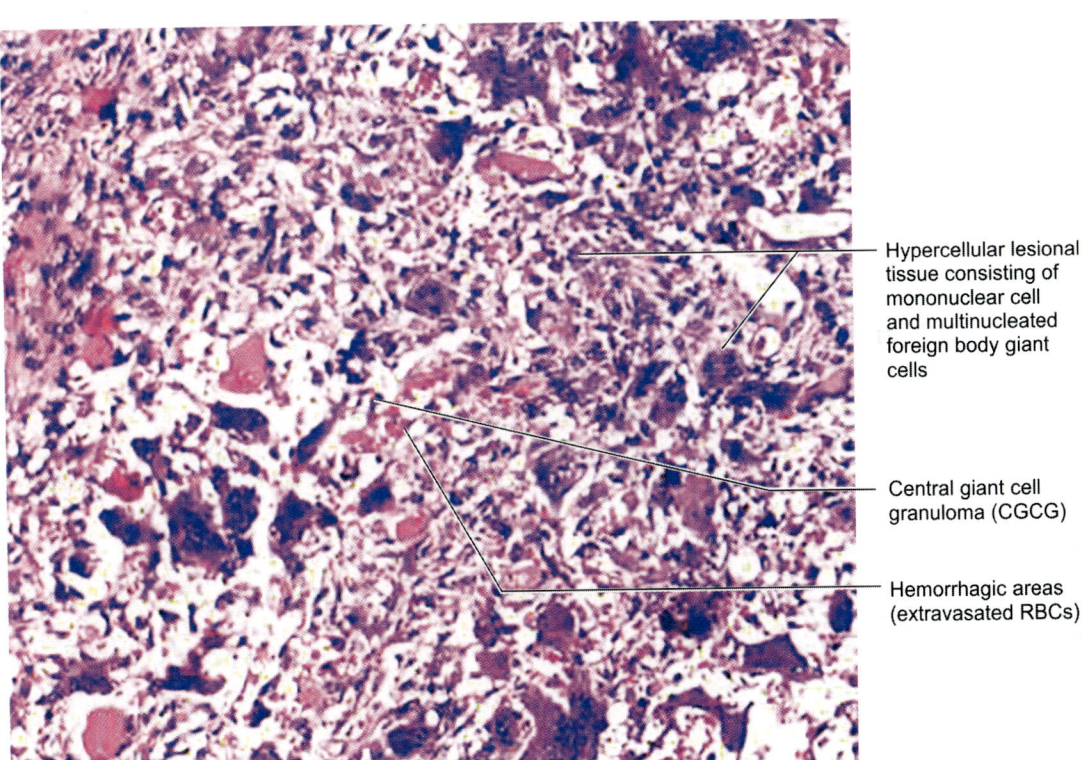

Hypercellular lesional tissue consisting of mononuclear cell and multinucleated foreign body giant cells

Central giant cell granuloma (CGCG)

Hemorrhagic areas (extravasated RBCs)

Fig. 4.1: 10X

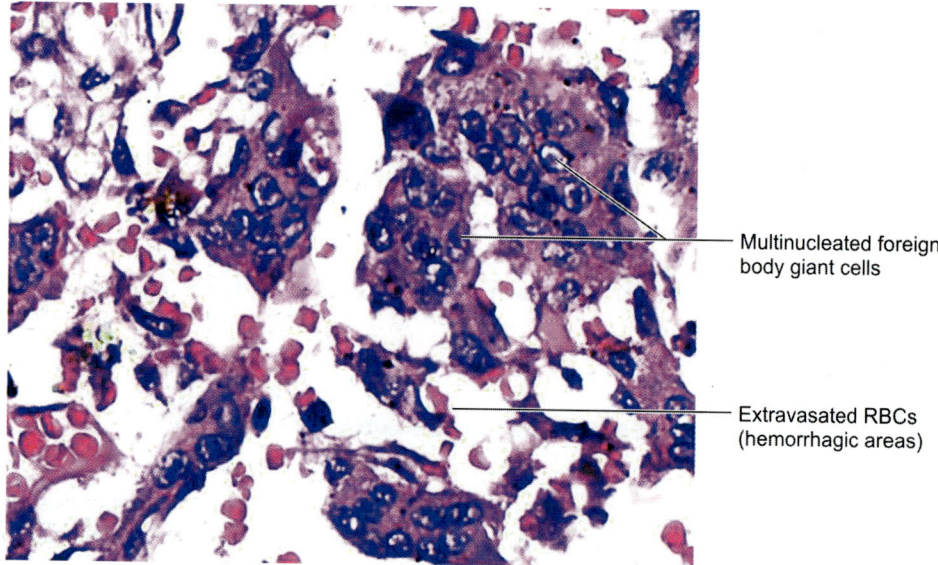

Multinucleated foreign body giant cells

Extravasated RBCs (hemorrhagic areas)

Fig. 4.2: 40X

Key Points

- Central giant cell granuloma (CGCG) is an uncommon reactive and proliferative lesion whose etiology is not defined.
- It was Jaffe who first introduced the term central giant cell reparative granuloma to distinguish this lesion from the giant cell tumor of long bones.
- However, since a reparative response was quite rare and most of these lesions were found to be destructive rather than reparative, the word reparative was omitted from that term.
- CGCG may be seen in all age groups, it is much more common in the younger individuals under 30 years of age.
- Females more commonly affected than males.
- Two-thirds of these cases occur in the mandible, and only one-third in the maxilla.
- Lesions are more common in the anterior segments of the jaws and usually cross the midline.
- Depending on clinical and radiographic features, CGCG can be classified into two types: Aggressive and non-aggressive.

Radiographic Appearance

Radiolucent area with either a relatively smooth or a ragged border.

Histopathological Picture

- Hypercellular lesional tissue consisting of mononuclear cells with multinucleated giant cells.
- Groups of collagen fibers are often arranged in whorled appearance.
- The giant cells vary in size from case to case and may contain few to several dozens of nuclei.
- In addition, there are usually numerous foci of old extravasated blood and associated hemosiderin pigment, some of it phagocytized by macrophages.
- Foci of new trabeculae of osteoid or bone also are often seen, particularly around the periphery of the lesion.

Additional Point

Rule out brown tumor (hyperparathyroidism).

GIANT CELL

Introduction

- Giant cells are called giant cells because of their unusual large size. They can be either uninucleated or multinucleated.
- Giant cells can be physiological or pathological. Physiological ones are odontoclast, megakaryocyte, osteoclast and pathological are foreign body type, Langhans' type, Reed-Sternberg giant cell, touton type giant cells, etc.
- Multinucleated giant cells (MGCs) are formed from the fusion of monocyte/macrophage.
- MGCs phenotypes vary, depending on the local environment, the chemical and physical (size) nature of the agent to which the MGCs and their monocyte/macrophage precursors are responding.

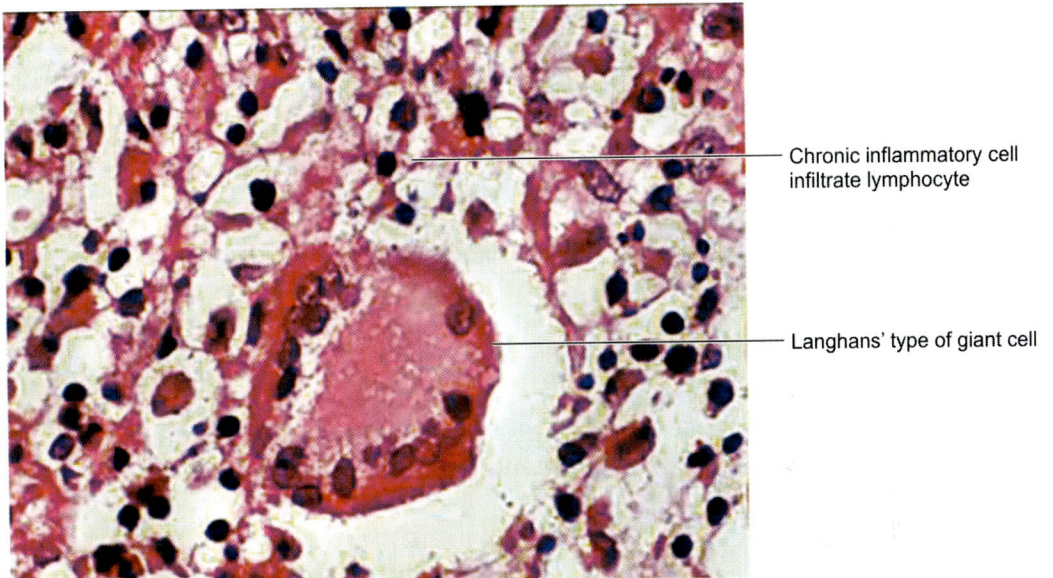

Chronic inflammatory cell infiltrate lymphocyte

Langhans' type of giant cell

Fig. 4.3: 40X Langhans' type giant cell

Key Points

- Langhans' type giant cells are found in granulomatous conditions (TB, leprosy, sarcoidosis, chelitis granulomatosa).
- They are formed by the fusion of epithelioid cells (modified macrophages), and contain nuclei arranged in a horseshoe-shaped pattern in the cell periphery or at two poles of cell.
- Center of giant cell contains necrotic debris.
- Located in vicinity of small caseous areas or at edge of larger areas.

REED STERNBERG CELL

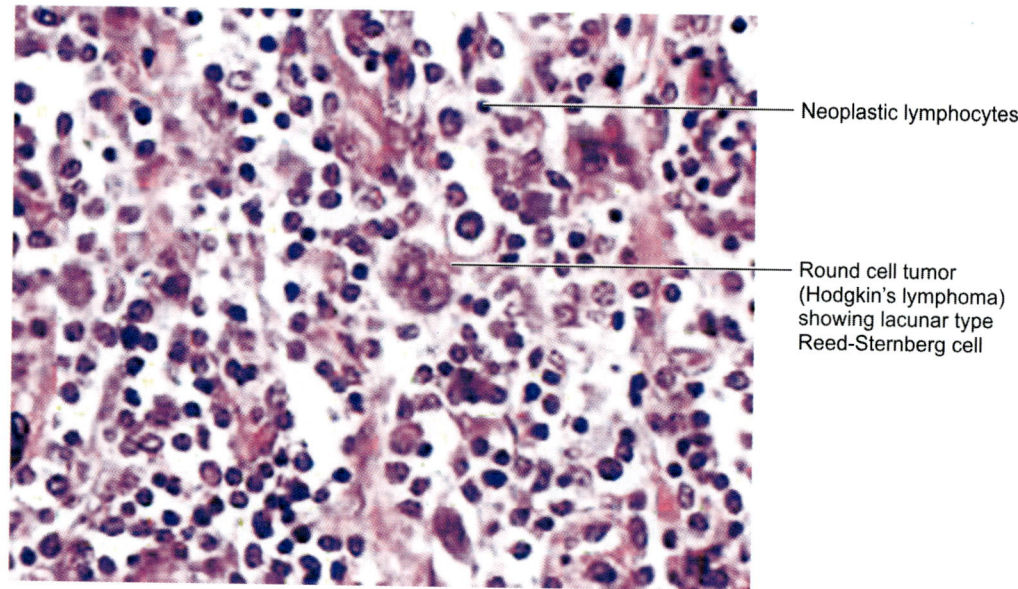

Neoplastic lymphocytes

Round cell tumor (Hodgkin's lymphoma) showing lacunar type Reed-Sternberg cell

Fig. 4.4: 40X

Key Points

- Reed-Sternberg (RS) cells are pathologic giant cells.
- Pathognomic for Hodgkin's lymphoma.
- Different histologic subtypes of Hodgkin's disease (HD) shows different morphologic types of Reed-Sternberg cell. Classic RS cell, lacunar type RS cell, polyploid type (or popcorn type, pleomorphic RS cells.

Histopathological Picture

- Histopathologically RS cell is a very large cell (15 to 45 um in diameter) with an multilobate nucleus, prominent nucleoli and abundant, usually slightly eosinophilic cytoplasm.
- Particular characteristic feature is cells with two mirror—image nuclei or nuclear lobes, each containing a large (inclusion-like) acidophilic nucleolus surrounded by a clear zone, features that impart an owl-eye appearance.

ACTINOMYCOSIS

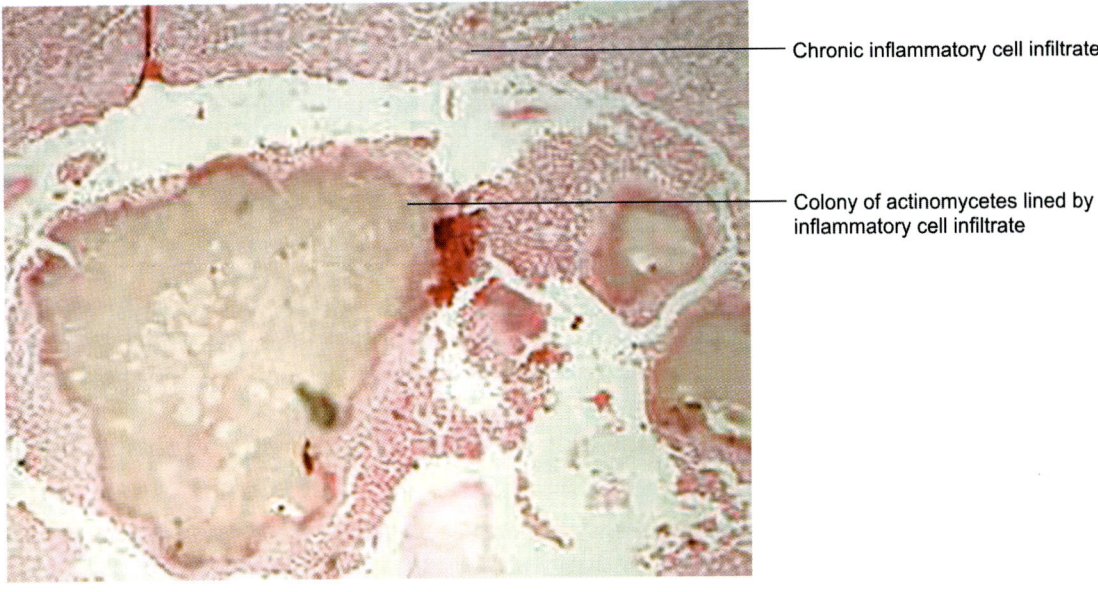

— Chronic inflammatory cell infiltrate

— Colony of actinomycetes lined by inflammatory cell infiltrate

Fig. 4.5: 4X

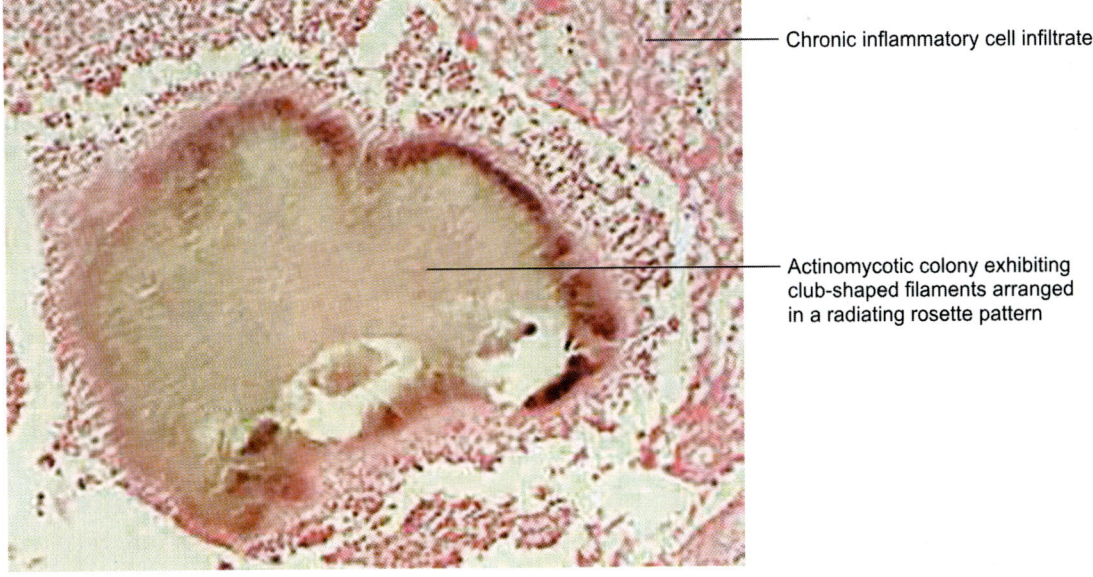

— Chronic inflammatory cell infiltrate

— Actinomycotic colony exhibiting club-shaped filaments arranged in a radiating rosette pattern

Fig. 4.6: 10X

Key Points

- Chronic granulomatous suppurative and fibrosing disease caused by anaerobic or microaerophilic gram-positive non-acid fast, branched filamentous bacteria.
- Most of the species isolated from actinomycotic lesions have been identified as *Actinomyces israelii, A. viscosus, A. odontolyticus, A. naeslundii or A meyeri.*
- Types are cervicofacial (most common), abdominal, pulmonary forms.
- Formation of abscesses that tend to drain by the formation of sinus tracts.
- If the pus from the abscess is examined on a clean glass slide, it shows the typical 'sulfur granules' or colonies of organisms.

Histopathological Picture

- Granulomatous lesion with central abscess formation and colonies of microorganisms. These colonies appear to be floating in a sea of polymorphonuclear leukocytes, often associated with multinucleated giant cells and macrophages particularly around the periphery of the lesion.
- With hematoxylin and eosin stains the central core stains basophilic and the peripheral portion is eosinophilic (ray fungus).

FOREIGN BODY GIANT CELL

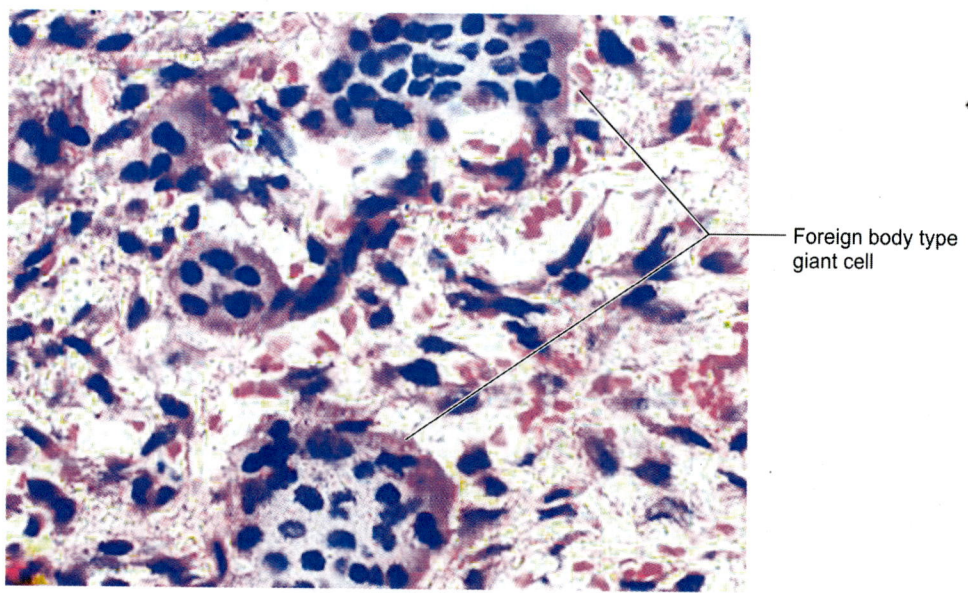

Foreign body type giant cell

Fig. 4.7: 40X

Key Points

- A foreign-body giant cell is a collection of fused macrophages (giant cell) which are generated in response to the presence of a large foreign body.
- The nuclei are arranged in a disorganized manner.
- The nuclei in this cell are centrally placed and overlap each other.
- Seen in PGCG, CGCG.

OSTEOMYELITIS

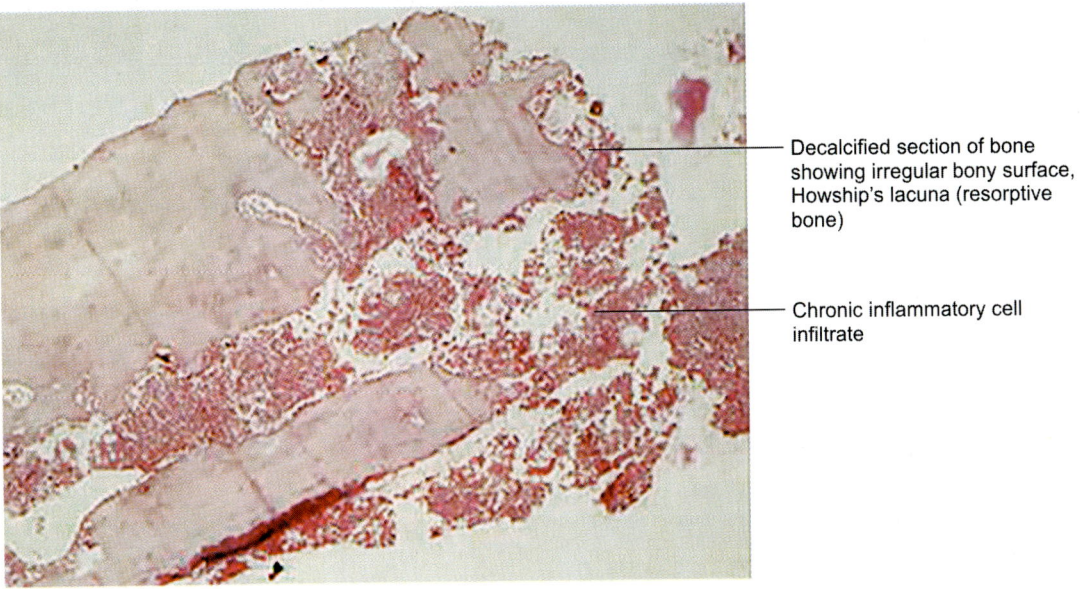

Decalcified section of bone showing irregular bony surface, Howship's lacuna (resorptive bone)

Chronic inflammatory cell infiltrate

Fig. 4.8: 10X

Key Points

- Osteomyelitis Greek word (*osteo*= bone, *muelion*= marrow, *itis* = inflammation) 'An inflammation of the medullary portion of bone'.
- Osteomyelitis is an 'inflammatory condition of bone that begins as an infection of the medullary cavity and haversian system and extends to involve the periosteum of the affected area'.
- Osteomyelitis of the mandible is much more frequent than that of maxilla
  a. Blood supply (maxilla has collateral blood supply).
  b. Cortical plates and medullary tissues.
  c. Boundaries.
  d. Traumatic incidents.
- Radiographic: Radiolucent appearance with irregular bony margin.
- 'Moth-eaten' appearance because of enlargement of medullary spaces and widening of Volkmann's canals secondary to destruction by lysis and replacement with granulation tissue.

Histopathological Picture

- Acute and chronic OML encompasses the full scope of inflammatory infiltrates ranging from mainly inflammatory exudate composed of fibrin, PMNs and macrophages.
- Bony tissue shows necrotic changes consisting of loss of the osteocytes from their lacunae, peripheral irregular bony surface with Howship's lacunae.
- Dead bone is called 'sequestra' and new bone is called 'involucrum'.
- Cloacae are the draining sinus/perforation from new bone.

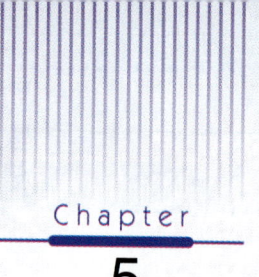

Connective Tissue Tumors

LIPOMA

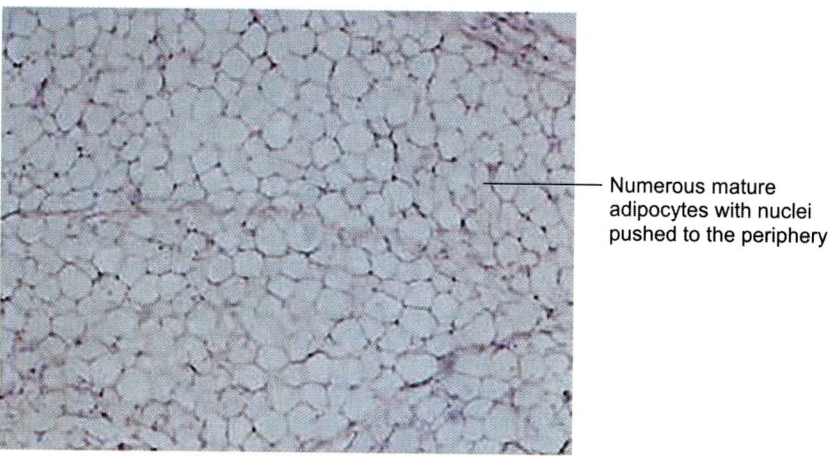

Numerous mature adipocytes with nuclei pushed to the periphery

Fig. 5.1: 4X

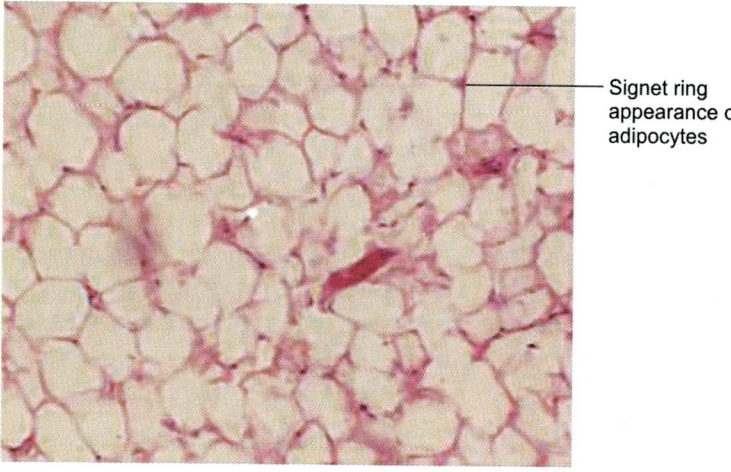

Signet ring appearance of adipocytes

Fig. 5.2: 10X

Key Points

- Relatively a rare intraoral, slow-growing neoplasm composed of mature fat cells.
- Usually found in adults and there is no gender predilection.
- The buccal mucosa, tongue, and floor of the mouth are among the common locations.
- Depending upon thinness of overlying epithelium the yellow coloration of fat can be seen and well-encapsulated, lipoma are freely movable beneath the mucosa.
- Gross specimen of lipoma is yellowish, relatively soft to palpation and has greasy (slippery) surface.
- Multiple head and neck lipomas have been observed in neurofibromatosis, Gardner's syndrome, encephalocraniocutaneous lipomatosis, multiple familial lipomatosis, and proteus syndrome.

Histopathological Picture

- The lipoma is composed predominantly of mature adipocytes, possibly admixed with collagenic streaks, and is often well-demarcated from the surrounding connective tissues by capsule.
- Tumor cells show nucleus pushed toward the cytoplasmic membrane (signet-ring appearance).

Additional Point

The excised tissue specimen floats in formalin.

OSTEOMA

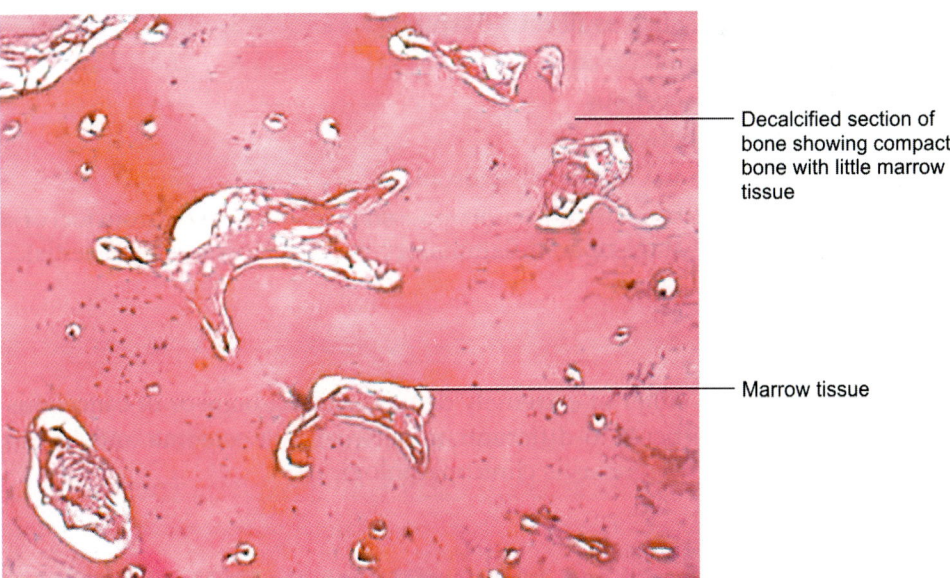

Decalcified section of bone showing compact bone with little marrow tissue

Marrow tissue

Fig. 5.3: 4X

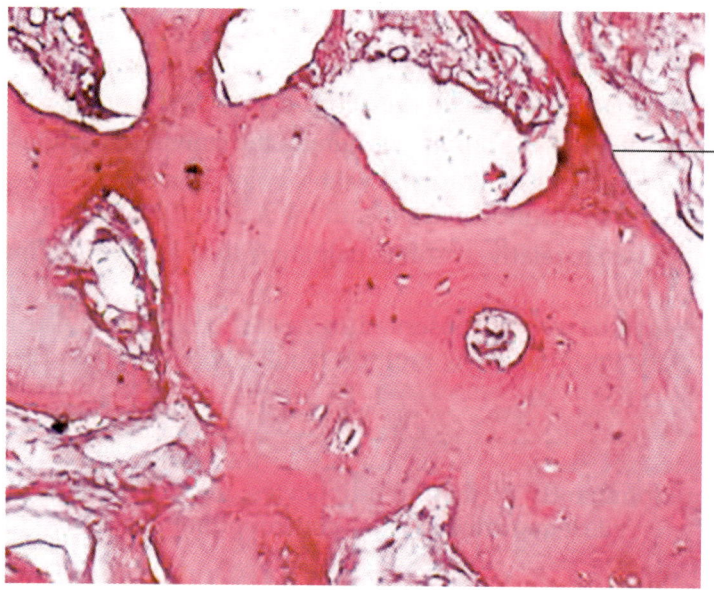

Decalcified section of bone showing compact bone with marrow tissue

Fig. 5.4: 10X

Key Points

- Benign, slow growing neoplasm usually asymptomatic.
- Can occur at any age, but common in adults.
- There is some question as to whether osteomas represent true neoplasms or a reactive lesion. Some likely represent the end stage of an injury or inflammatory process or the end stage of a hamartomatous process, such as fibrous dysplasia.
- Mandible more commonly involved.
- Two types—compact or cancellous
- Central or subperiosteal (peripheral)
- Multiple osteoma are seen in Gardner's syndrome.
- Smaller endosteal osteomas are difficult, if not impossible to differentiate from foci of sclerotic bone representing the end stage of an inflammatory process (condensing osteitis).

Histopathological Picture

- Compact or cancellous.
- The osteoma is composed either of extremely dense, compact bone or of cancellous bone.
- In any given area it is difficult to differentiate between the osteoma and normal bone histopathologically alone (diagnosis is clinicopathological).

Additional Point

Tori, exostosis, bony excrescence and even normal bone can be confused with osteoma histopathologically.

FIBROSARCOMA

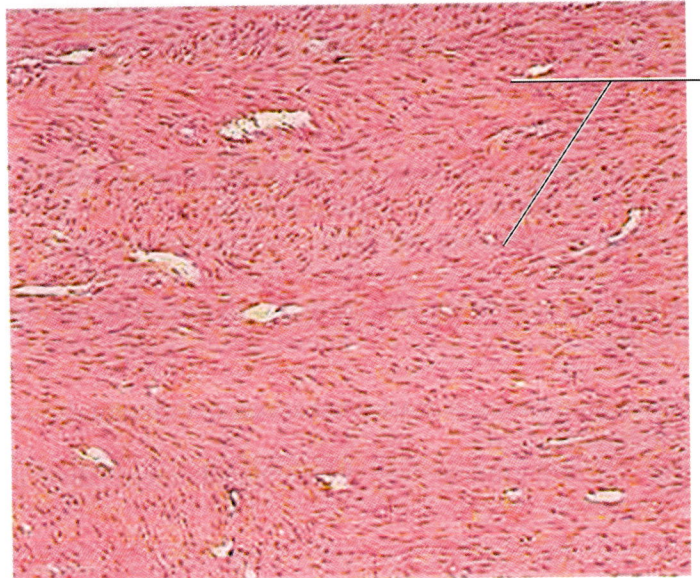

Hypercellular lesional tissue consisting of fibroblastic proliferation showing herring bone pattern

Fig. 5.5: 10X

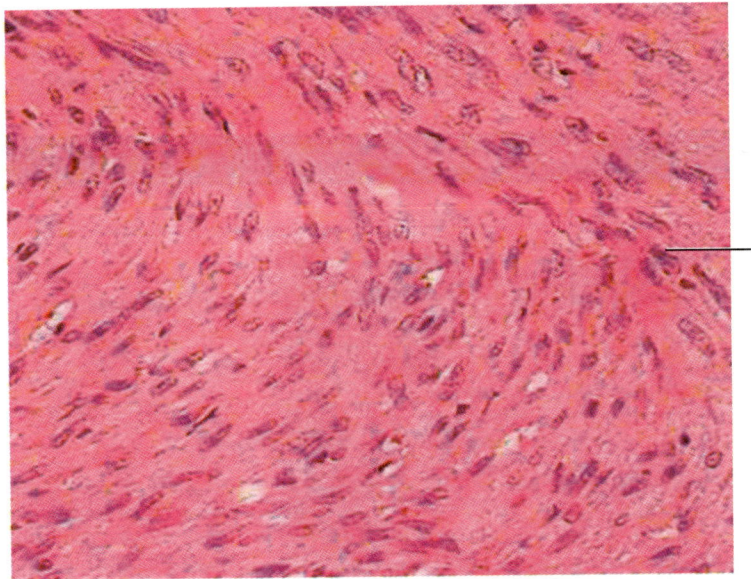

Neoplastic fibroblasts showing vesiculated nuclei

Fig. 5.6: 40X

Key Points

- Malignant mesenchymal neoplasm of fibroblasts that rarely affects the oral cavity.
- Fibrosarcoma of head and neck area represents 5% of all malignant intraosseous tumors.
- It can occur in any location, but mainly affects long bones particularly, and its occurrence in craniofacial region is about 15%, mandible being the most common site.
- Although fibrosarcoma has been reported in all groups, it is predominantly seen in the 3rd and 6th decade of life.

- Fibrosarcoma of bone has slight male predilection.
- The patient classically presents with pain, with or without swelling. In the oral cavity, mobility of teeth may be apparent.
- It has been reported in association with several conditions, such as Paget's disease, fibrous dysplasia and post-radiotherapy.

Histopathological Picture

- The classical fibrosarcoma has been characterized microscopically by uniform spindle cells distributed in interlacing fascicles with herring bone growth pattern.
- On high power view spindle cell shows cigar-shaped nuclei (not pathognomic as seen in other spindle cell lesions).
- Characteristically, the cells are uniform spindle-shaped (spindle cell sarcoma), multipolar, with elongated oval or round hyperchromatic nuclei and sometimes may vary little in size and shape.
- These cells are arranged in interlocking bands or fascicles that run in different directions, and may be arranged in a herringbone pattern.
- Histopathologically shows three different grades—well differentiated, intermediate grade and high grade.

Additional Points

- Differential diagnosis should include reactive fibromatosis, fibroblastic osteogenic sarcoma.
- The treatment of choice is surgical resection with a wide margin.
- The overall survival rate at 10 years may vary from 21.8 to 83%, and clinical stage, histological grade of malignancy, and local recurrences are the most important prognostic factors.

OSTEOSARCOMA

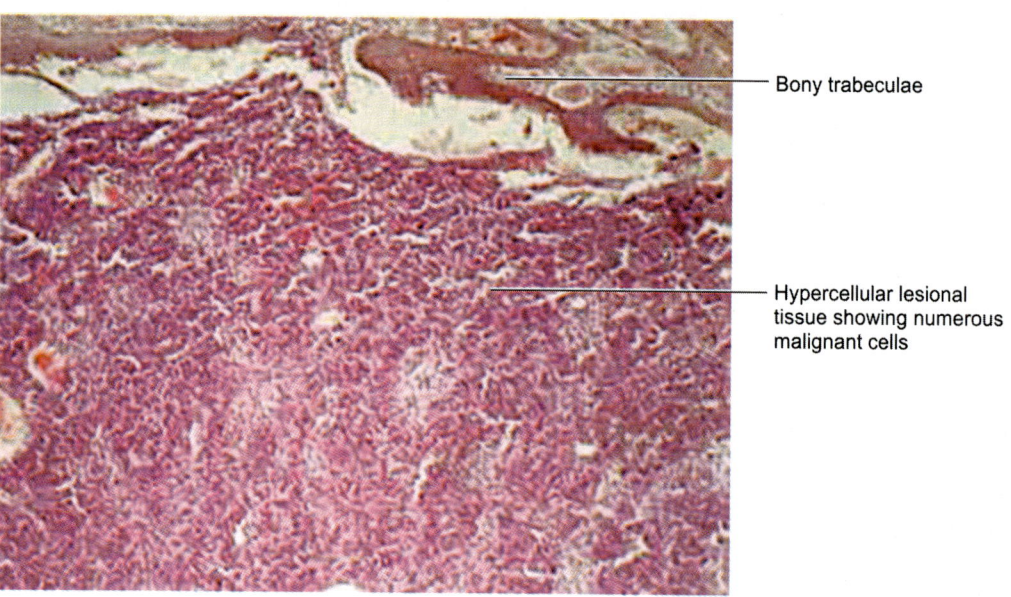

Bony trabeculae

Hypercellular lesional tissue showing numerous malignant cells

Fig. 5.7: 4X

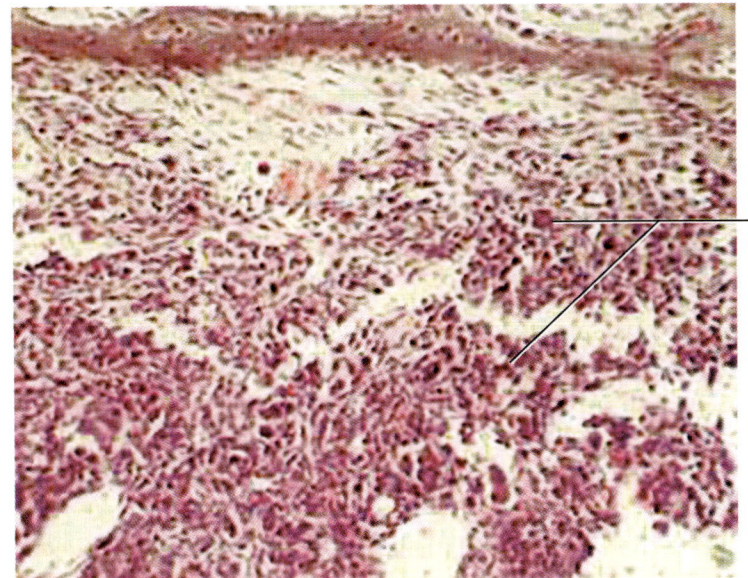

Round to ovoid hyperchromatic malignant cells with anaplastic giant cells

Fig. 5.8: 10X

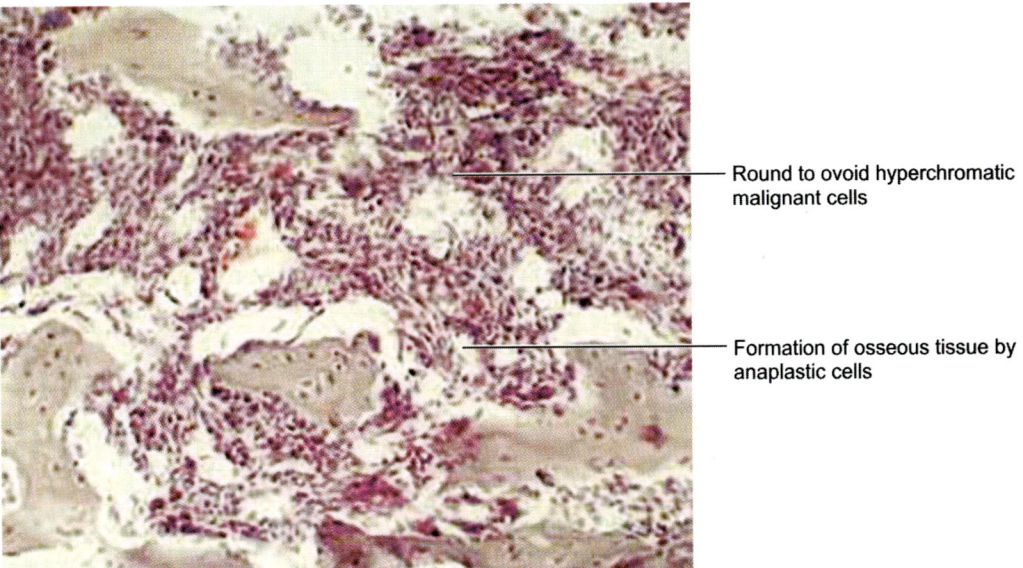

Round to ovoid hyperchromatic malignant cells

Formation of osseous tissue by anaplastic cells

Fig. 5.9: 10X

Key Points

- Common primary malignant tumor of the bone.
- Characterized by formation of osteoid or bone, or both, directly by sarcoma cells.
- Thought to arise from primitive osteoblast-forming mesenchyme.
- Classified into two main categories: Central (medullary) and surface (parosteal and perosteal).
- Osteosarcomas of the jaws are uncommon.
- Mean age is about 33 years which is 10 to 15 years older than the counterpart seen in long bones.

Radiographic Features

- Varies from dense sclerotic to mixed sclerotic and radiolucent lesion.
- Small streaks of bone radiate outward from approximately 25% of these tumors. This produces a sunray (sunburst). Codman's triangle appearance is usually seen in long bones osteosarcoma (elevation of cortex).
- When tumor grows in the periodontal ligament space, resorption of the adjacent bone resulting in uniform widening of the PDL space is noted.

Histopathological Picture

- Histopathologically osteosarcoma shows hypercellular lesional tissue composed of hyperchromatic, round or spindle-shaped cells to highly pleomorphic cells with bizarre nucleus.
- The neoplastic cells show varying degree of differentiation.
- The characteristic feature is direct production of osteoid (malignant osteoid) and bone by malignant mesenchymal cells.
- In addition to osteoid and bone, the tumor cells may produce fibrous tissue, myxoid tissue or cartilage.
- Differential diagnosis include round cell and spindle cell lesions, e.g. rhabdomyosarcoma, leiomyosarcoma, aggressive ostoblastoma, chondrosarcoma.

Salivary Gland Lesions

MUCOCELE

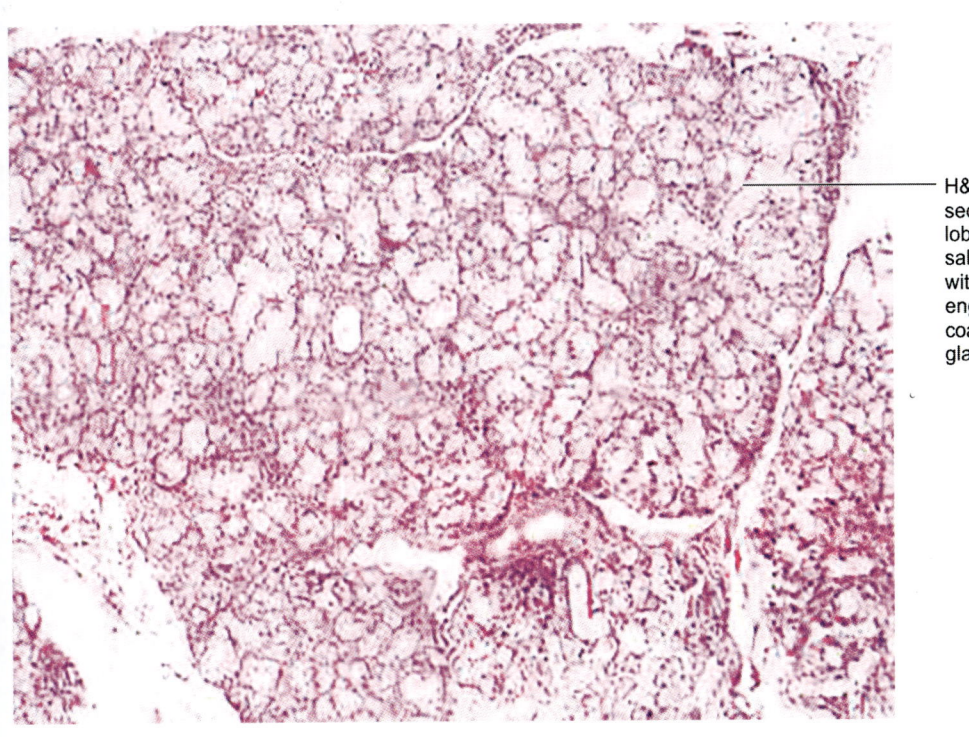

H&E stain section showing lobules of salivary gland with numerous engorged and coalesced salivary gland acini

Fig. 6.1: 4X

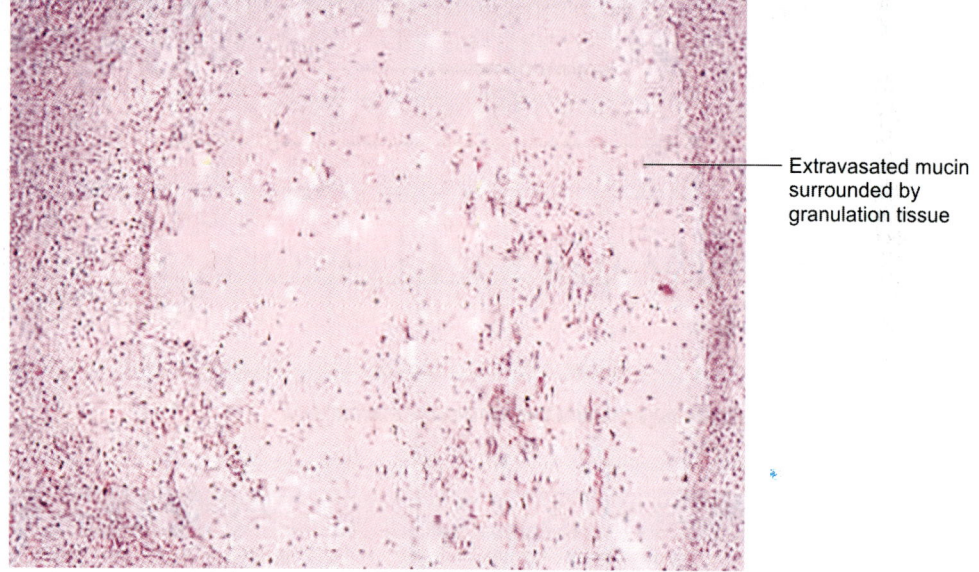

Extravasated mucin surrounded by granulation tissue

Fig. 6.2: 10X

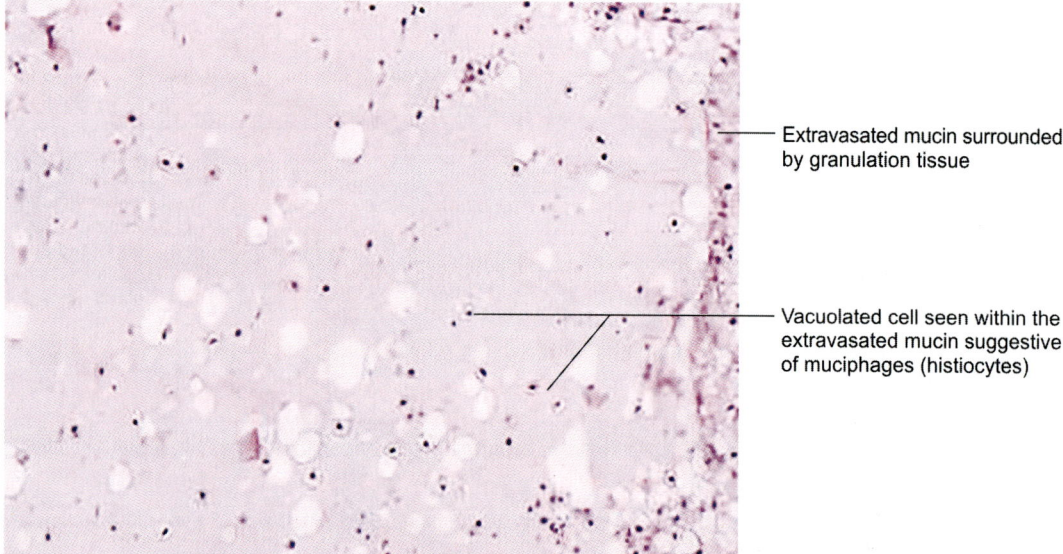

Extravasated mucin surrounded by granulation tissue

Vacuolated cell seen within the extravasated mucin suggestive of muciphages (histiocytes)

Fig. 6.3: 10X

Key Points

- Etiology: Trauma and obstruction of salivary gland ducts.
- The lower lip is the most frequent site because of trauma.
- Two histological types exist-extravasation and retention type.

- Clinically present as a soft, bluish or transparent cystic swelling which normally resolves spontaneously.
- The blue color is caused by vascular congestion, cyanosis and the accumulation of mucin.

Histopathological Picture

- Histopathologic picture shows numerous engorged salivary gland acini; coalescing of acini with spilled eosinophilic material suggestive of mucin.
- Extravasated mucin seen lined by granulation tissue with diffuse areas of chronic inflammatory cell infiltrates.
- Vacuolated cells seen within the extravasated mucin suggestive of muciphages (histiocytes).

Additional Points

- The term ranula is used to denote mucocele of floor of mouth.
- Ranula word is derived from latin rana word mean frog because swelling resemble translucent underbelly of frog (Rana Tigrina).
- An unusual clinical variant is plunging or cervical ranula, where the swelling is in the neck rather than the floor of the mouth.
- Clinical differential diagnosis include lipoma of the lip (depending upon location).

PLEOMORPHIC ADENOMA (PA)

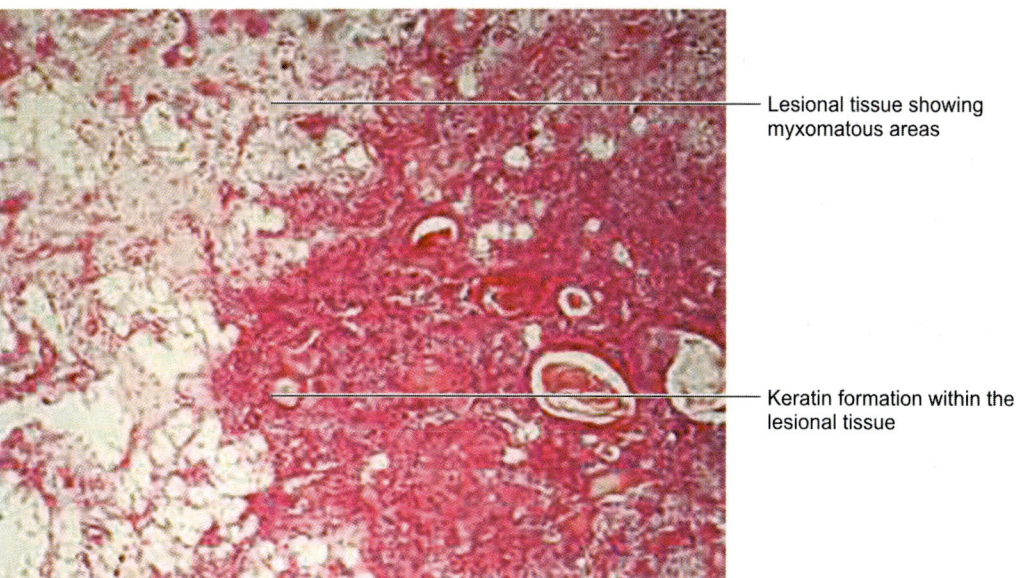

Lesional tissue showing myxomatous areas

Keratin formation within the lesional tissue

Fig. 6.4: 4X

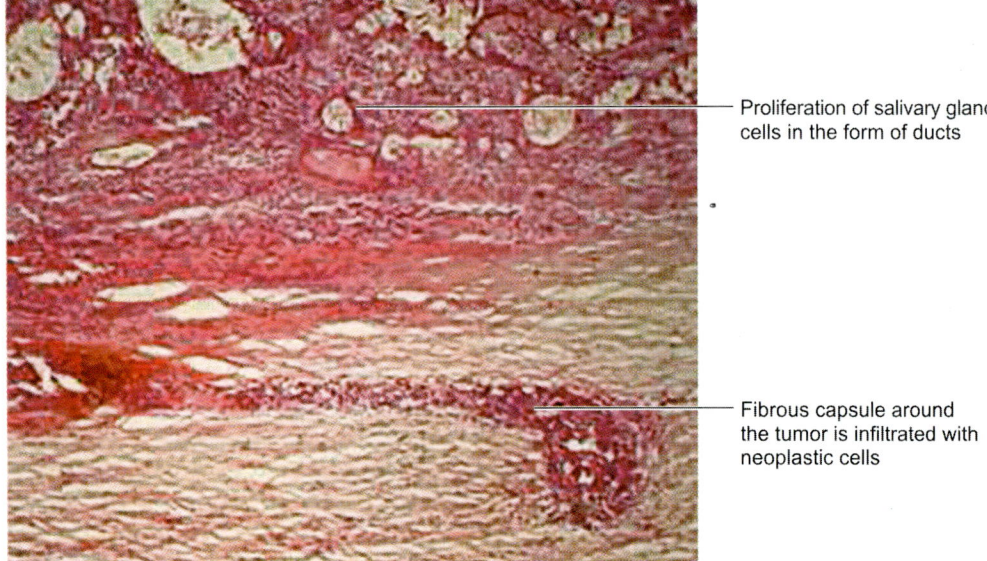

Proliferation of salivary gland cells in the form of ducts

Fibrous capsule around the tumor is infiltrated with neoplastic cells

Fig. 6.5: 4X

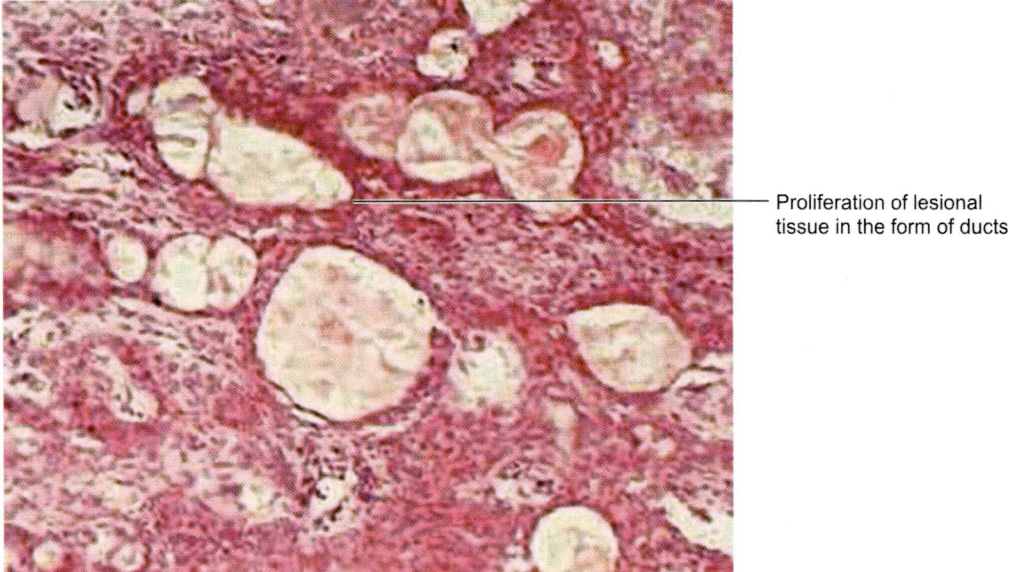

Proliferation of lesional tissue in the form of ducts

Fig. 6.6: 10X

Key Points

- Benign epithelial salivary gland tumor.
- Most common tumor of the salivary glands.
- Synonyms used is mixed tumor, although a misnomer.
- Mostly seen in 4th–6th decade of life with female predilection (F : M–6 : 4).
- Parotid gland and palate are the most common site involved for major salivary and minor salivary glands respectively.
- The usual clinical presentation is a painless swelling.

Histopathological Picture

- Histopathologically, it is partially encapsulated, the fibrous capsule may be infiltrated by with tumor cells.
- Hallmark/characteristic of PA is chondromyxoid stroma.
- Two cell population, i.e. ductal cell and myoepithelial cell is seen.
- Neoplastic cells may be seen arranged in ductal pattern, sheets and islands.
- Various tissues are seen, like keratin, osseous tissue, chondroid tissue, fat tissue and myxoid tissue, etc.

WARTHIN TUMOR

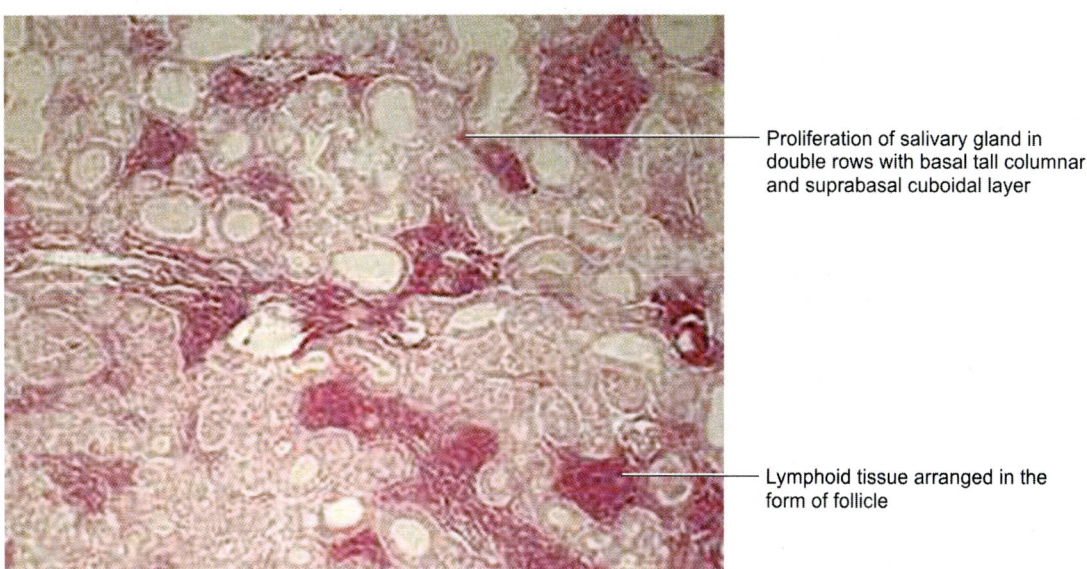

Proliferation of salivary gland in double rows with basal tall columnar and suprabasal cuboidal layer

Lymphoid tissue arranged in the form of follicle

Fig. 6.7: 4X

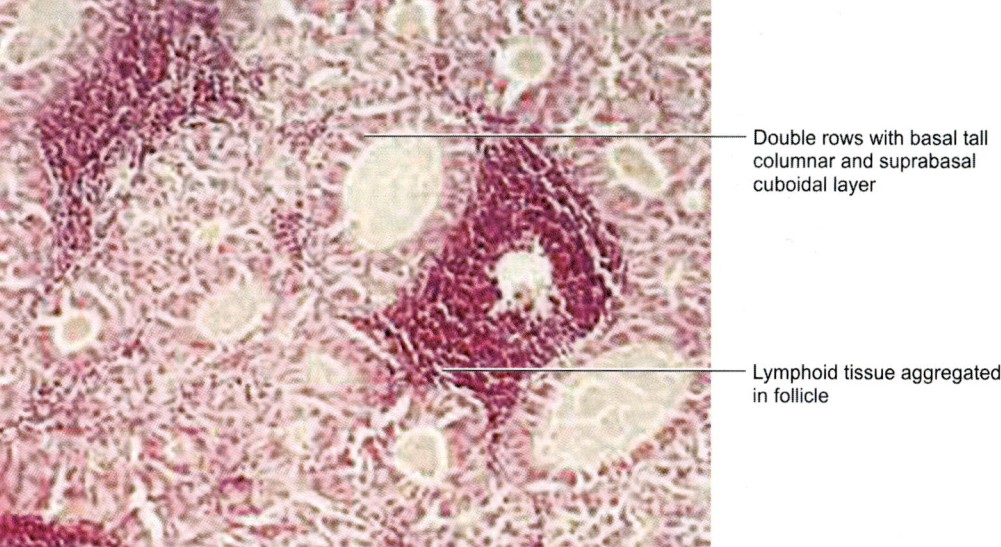

Double rows with basal tall columnar and suprabasal cuboidal layer

Lymphoid tissue aggregated in follicle

Fig. 6.8: 10X

Key Points

- Benign epithelial salivary gland tumor.
- Second most common tumor of salivary glands.
- Other names are papillary cystadenoma lymphomatosum, adenolymphoma.
- Mostly seen in the 6th and 7th decade of life with definite male predilection.
- Strong association with smoking.
- Common clinical presentation is painless swelling.

Histopathological Picture

- Histopathologically, two components are noted—epithelial and lymphoid tissue.
- Tumor shows papillary projections into the cystic spaces and lymphoid matrix showing germinal centers.
- The cyst are lined by papillary proliferations of bilayered oncocytic epithelium. The inner layer cells are tall columnar while outer cells are basaloid in appearance.
- Cystic spaces are filled with eosinophilic coagulum.

MUCOEPIDERMOID CARCINOMA (MEC)

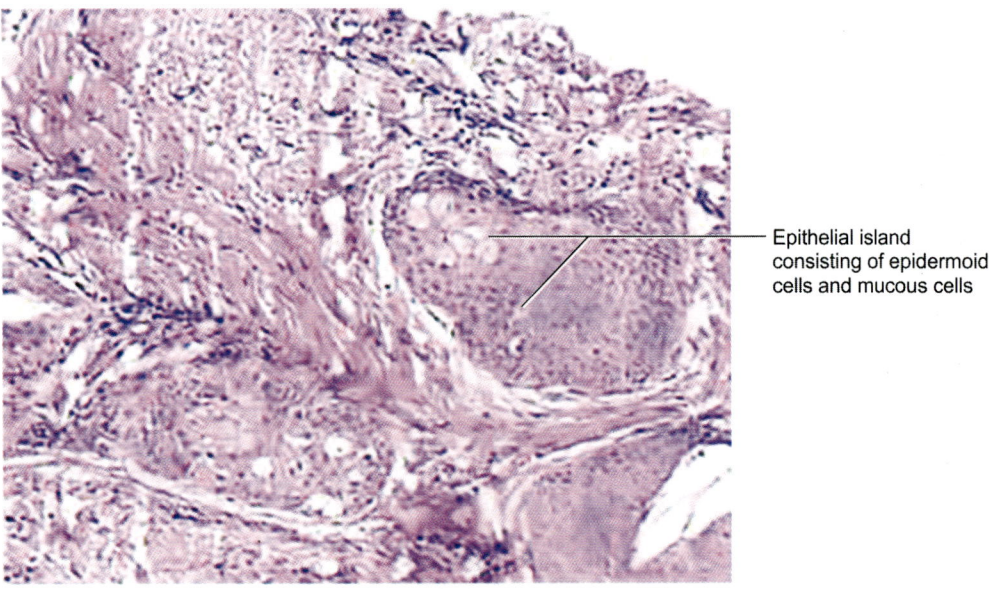

Epithelial island consisting of epidermoid cells and mucous cells

Fig. 6.9: 10X

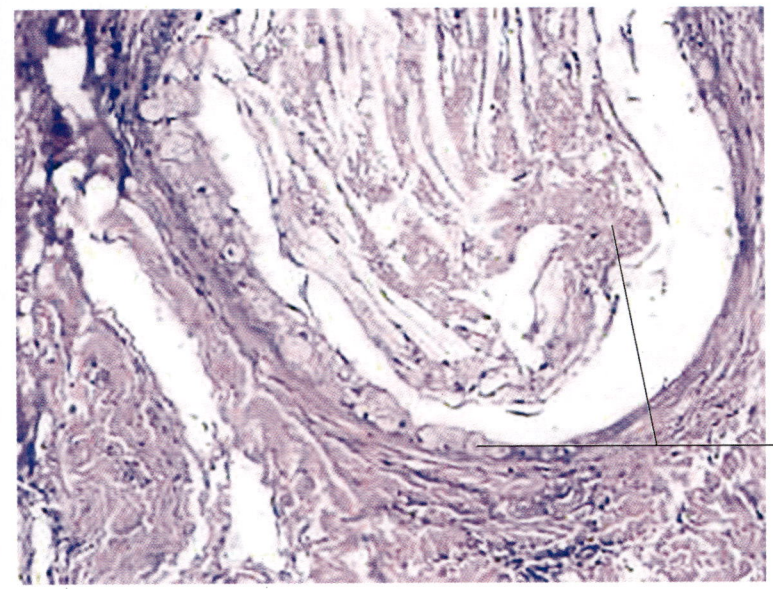

Microcyst-lining predominantly consist of mucous cells and lumen filled with degenerated and mucinous material

Fig. 6.10: 10X

Key Points

- Malignant salivary gland tumor.
- Occurs primarily in the third or fifth decade of life, with an average age of 47 years, with a slight female predilection.
- Among the major and minor salivary glands the parotid and palatal glands are the most common sites respectively
- Prior exposure to ionizing radiation appears to substantially increase the risk of developing mucoepidermoid carcinoma.
- The tumor of low-grade malignancy usually appears as a slowly enlarging, painless mass which simulates the pleomorphic adenoma.

Histopathological Picture

- Three histological variants—low, intermediate and high grade.
- Islands consisting of squamous epithelial cells along with cystic spaces and few mucous cells.
- From low to high grade the mucous cell and cystic component decreases while solid epithelial component increases.
- Low grade shows minimal pleomorphism, hyperchromatism and mitotic figures.
- As grade increases pleomorphism and mitotic activity increases.
- Keratin formation can also be seen.
- Mucoid like material is present in cystic spaces.

Additional Point

Intraosseous MEC can arise from odontogenic cysts (dentigerous cyst, glandular odontogenic cyst, etc.), entrapped salivary glands during development and maxillary sinus lining.

Fibro-osseous Lesion

FIBROUS DYSPLASIA

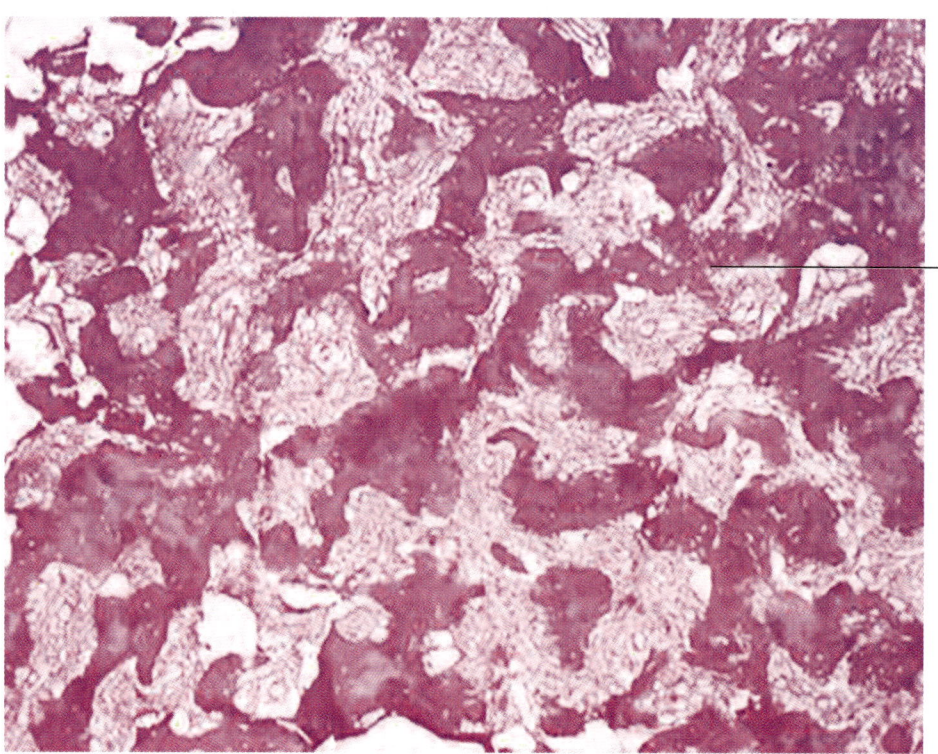

Lesional
tissue
consisting
of irregularly
shaped bony
trabeculae
within loose
fibrous stroma

Fig. 7.1: 4X

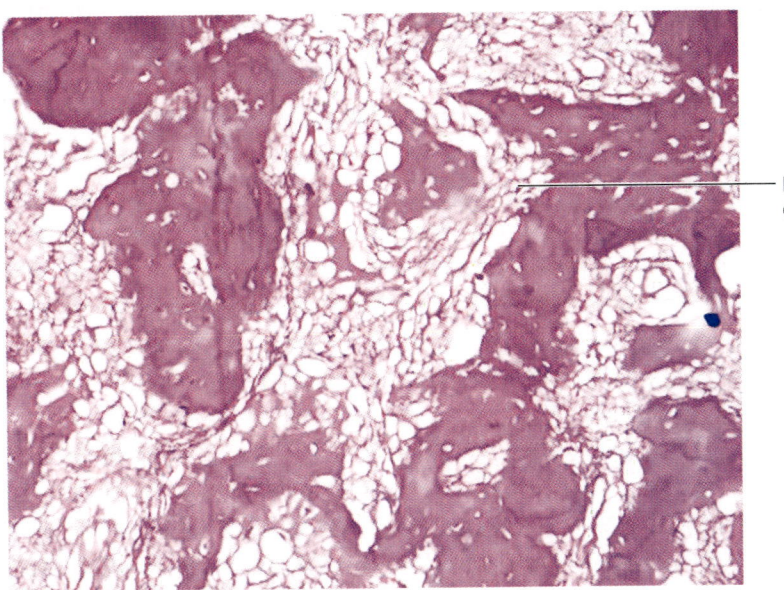

Bony trabeculae in delicate fibrillar stroma

Fig. 7.2: 10X

Key Points

- GNAS1 (guanine nucleotide binding protein, α-stimulating activity polypeptide) mutation full form.
- 10–25% of patients with the monostotic form and 50% with the polyostotic form.
- Occurs during 1st and 2nd decade.
- Common sites of involvement are frontal, sphenoid, maxillary and ethmoid bones.
- Painless swelling with facial asymmetry.
- Although mandibular lesions are truly monostotic, maxillary lesions often involve adjacent bones, such as the zygoma, sphenoid and occiput, and are not strictly monostotic. The designation of craniofacial fibrous dysplasia (FD) is appropriate for these lesions.

Important terms and points related to FD	
Monostotic	Single bone
Polyostotic	Multiple bones of the body
Craniofacial	Craniofacial bones
Jaffe's type	Polyostotic FD + skin pigmentation
McCune-Albright syndrome	Polyostotic FD + skin pigmentation + hyperfunctioning endocrinopathies
Mazabraud's syndrome	FD + intramuscular myxomas

Monostotic FD	Polyostotic FD
Single bone involved	Multiple bones involved
Absence of osteoblastic rim	Osteoblastic rim may be present, depends on—bone involved and stage of lesion
Dysplastic bone does not reach to lamellar pattern	Lamellar bone may be seen
Alkaline phosphatase level is normal	Alkaline phosphatase level raised at later stage

- Most malignant neoplasms develop in patients who previously have undergone radiation therapy to the affected area and common ones are osteosarcoma, followed by fibrosarcoma and chondrosarcoma.

Radiographic Appearance

'Orange Peel' appearance of fine dense trabeculae and ground glass (Frosted glass).

Histopathological Picture

Macroscopic

- Consistency → variable, soft to very hard.
- Color → grayish white tissue
- Gritty texture when cut with a scalpel
- Deformity of the affected bone is observed
- Microscopic: The typical microscopic findings of fibrous dysplasia show irregularly shaped trabeculae of immature (woven) bone in a cellular, loosely arranged fibrillar stroma.
- They often assume curvilinear shapes, which have been likened to chinese script writing.
- The bony trabeculae are considered to arise by metaplasia and are not usually surrounded by osteoid seams or plump appositional osteoblasts.
- The lesional bone fuses directly with normal bone at the periphery of the lesion, so that no capsule or line of demarcation is present.

OSSIFYING FIBROMA

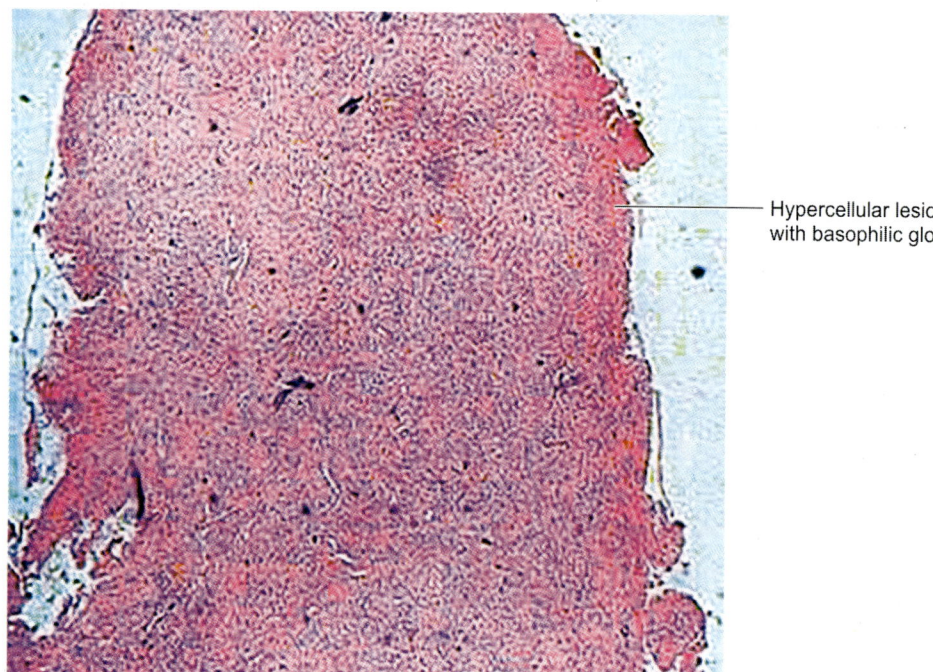

Hypercellular lesional tissue with basophilic globular areas

Fig. 7.3: 4X

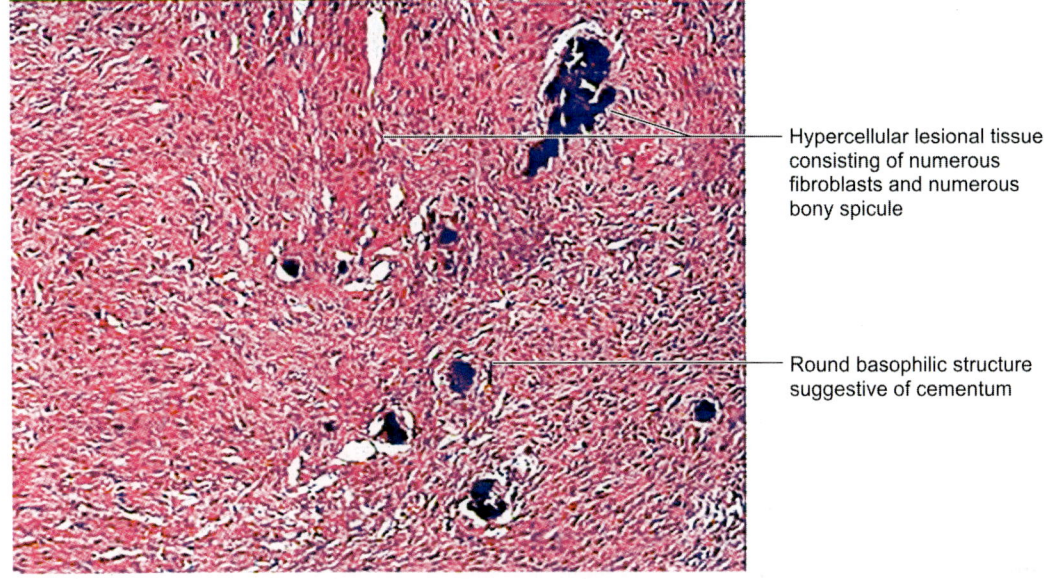

Hypercellular lesional tissue consisting of numerous fibroblasts and numerous bony spicule

Round basophilic structure suggestive of cementum

Fig. 7.4: 10X

Key Points

- Ossifying fibromas (OF) occur over a wide age range with the greatest number of cases encountered during the third and fourth decade of life.
- Definite female predilection, with mandible involved more often than the maxilla.
- The mandibular premolar and molar area is the most common site.
- Radiographic picture: OFs typically appear as unilocular lesions with sharply defined, smooth, corticated borders a feature that is used to differentiate OFs from FD.
- Radiographic picture varies from radiolucent to mixed to complete radio-opaque.
- A thin, radiolucent line, representing a fibrous capsule, may separate it from surrounding bone.

Histopathological Picture

- Microscopic patterns, depending on the stage of the lesion and the degree of calcification.
- OFs usually consist of a moderately cellular, relatively avascular, dense fibrous stroma.
- The cells appear spindle-shaped to ovoid and may be haphazardly arranged or organized in a vague storiform pattern.
- The nuclei are bland appearing and contain single, inconspicuous nucleoli. Focally scattered multinucleated giant cells may also be seen.
- The calcified material may consist of thin, irregularly shaped trabeculae of woven bone; scattered trabeculae of lamellar bone; deposits of basophilic staining, round or ovoid, cellular or acellular calcified deposits that have been likened to cementum; or any combination there of.

Additional Point

Juvenile trabecular ossifying fibroma histopathologically can be confused with osteosarcoma and fibrosarcoma.

FLORID CEMENTO-OSSEOUS DYSPLASIA (FCOD)

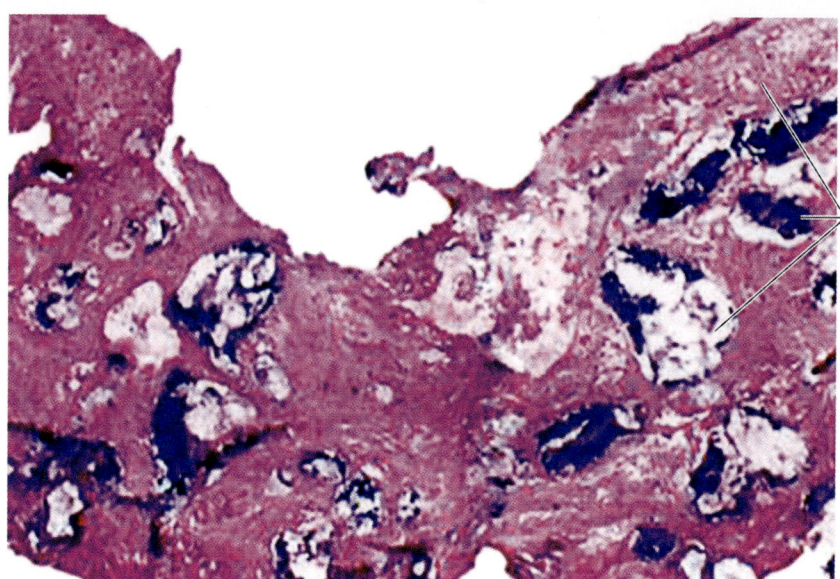

Decalcified section of lesional tissue consisting of fibrous connective tissue with numerous basophilic areas suggestive of cementum

Fig. 7.5a: 4X

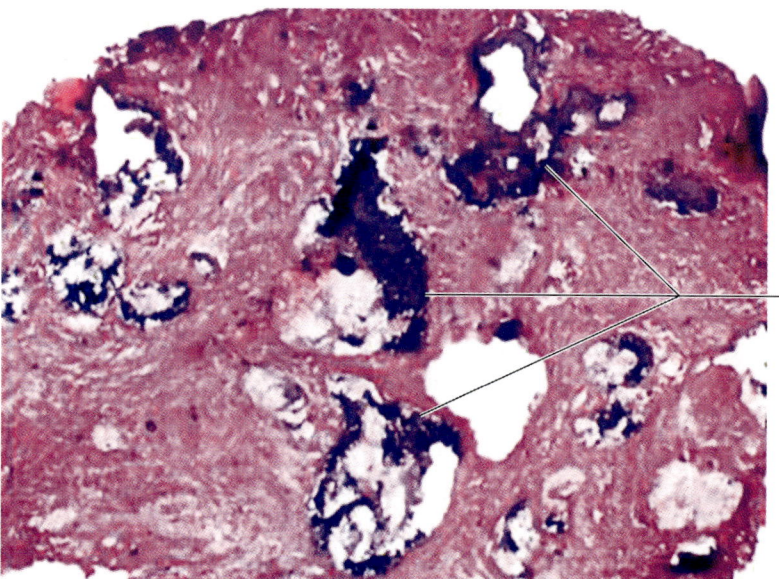

Decalcified section of lesional tissue consisting of fibrous connective tissue with numerous basophilic areas suggestive of cementum

Fig. 7.5b: 4X

Key Points

- Florid cemento-osseous dysplasia (FCOD) shows multifocal involvement not limited to the anterior mandible.
- Although many cases demonstrate multifocal lesions only in the posterior portions of the jaws, many patients also reveal synchronous involvement of the anterior mandible.

- The lesions show a marked tendency for bilateral and often quite symmetric involvement but extensive lesions in all four posterior quadrants can be seen.
- FCOD is more commonly seen in middle-aged black women, although it also may occur in Caucasians and Asians. In some cases, a familial trend can be observed.
- Usually asymptomatic and discovered only when radiographs are taken for some other purpose.
- The epicenter is apical to the teeth, within the alveolar process and usually posterior to the cuspid. In the mandible, lesions occur above the inferior alveolar canal.

Radiographic Picture

Depending upon the stage, radiographic picture varies from radiolucent to mixed to radio-opaque.

Histopathological Picture

- Florid cemento-osseous dysplasia is composed of fibrous connective tissue background with a mixture of woven bone, lamellar bone and cementum like areas.
- The proportion of each mineralized material varies from lesion to lesion and from area to area in individual sites of involvement. Irregular and round deposits of metaplastically formed 'cementoid' shows dark purple boundries and may seems fused, creating large globular masses. These coalescence impart a 'pagetoid' appearance.
- As the lesions mature and become more sclerotic, the ratio of fibrous connective tissue to mineralized material decreases.
- With progression to the final radio-opaque stage, individual trabeculae fuse and form lobular masses composed of sheets or fused globules of relatively acellular and disorganized cemento-osseous material.
- Once lesions become sclerotic they tend to become hypovascular and prone to necrosis, often minimal provocation can lead to osteomyelitis.

Additional Points

- Focal cemento-osseous dysplasia exhibits single site of involvement.
- Periapical cemento-osseous dysplasia predominantly involves the periapical region of anterior mandible.
- Differential diagnosis include condensing osteitis.

Potentially Premalignant Oral Epithelial Lesions (PPOELs)

LEUKOPLAKIA

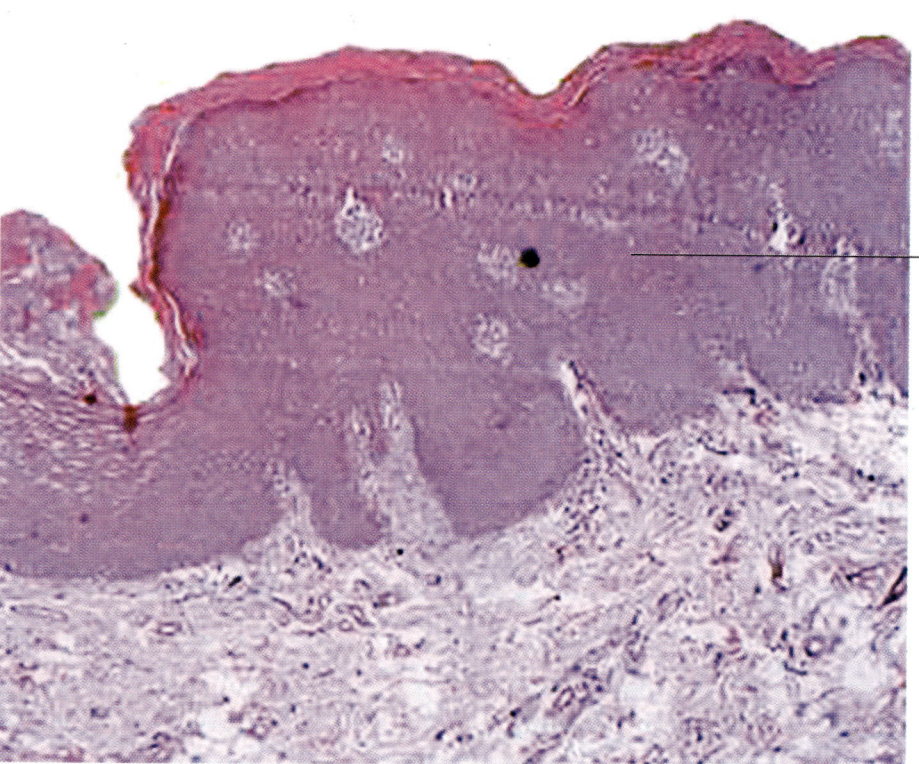

Proliferative hyper-parakeratotic stratified squamous epithelium with acanthosis and underlying fibrocellular connective tissue stroma

Fig. 8.1: 4X

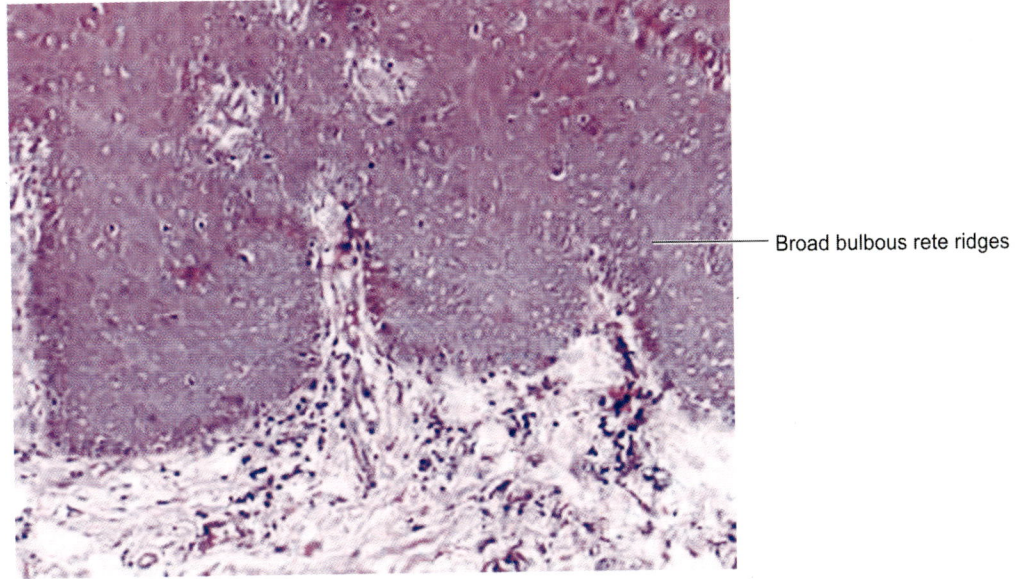

Broad bulbous rete ridges

Fig. 8.2: 10X

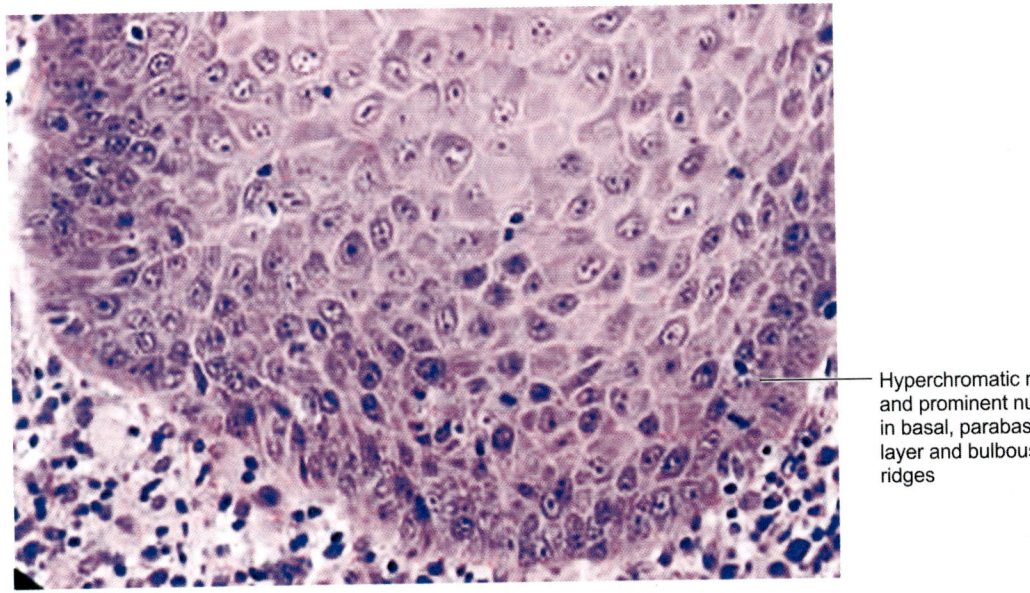

Hyperchromatic nuclei and prominent nucleoli in basal, parabasal cell layer and bulbous rete ridges

Fig. 8.3: 40X

Key Points

- The word dysplasia is derived from Latin dys – bad + Gr. Plassen – to form.
- Dysplasia means abnormal, atypical proliferation. Dysplasia is defined as architectural disturbance, accompanied by cytological atypia.
- Epithelial dysplasia is defined as 'a precancerous lesion of stratified squamous epithelium characterised by cellular atypia and loss of normal maturation and stratification short of carcinoma *in situ*' Pindborg et al (1997).

- According to the WHO classification (2005) several cellular and architectural changes in the epithelium have to be taken into consideration to report the lesion as dysplasia which are as follows:

Architectural (Tissue Changes)

- Irregular epithelial stratification.
- Loss of polarity of basal cells.
- Basal cell hyperplasia.
- Drop-shaped rete pegs.
- Increased number of mitotic figures.
- Abnormally superficial mitoses.
- Dyskeratosis (premature keratinization in single cells).
- Keratin pearls within rete ridges.

Cellular Changes

- Abnormal variation in nuclear size and shape (anisonucleosis and nuclear pleomorphism).
- Abnormal variation in cell size and shape (anisocytosis and cellular pleomorphism).
- Increased nuclear/cytoplasmic ratio.
- Enlarged nuclei.
- Atypical mitotic figures.
- Increased number and size of nucleoli.
- Hyperchromasia.

VERRUCOUS HYPERPLASIA

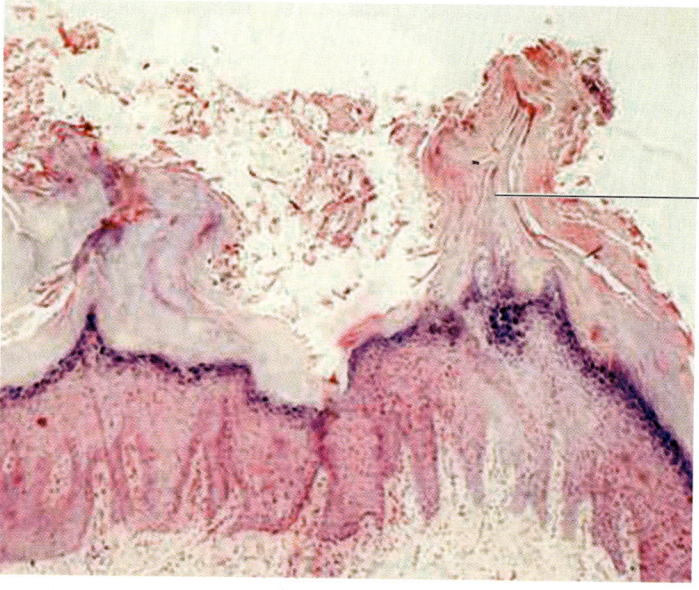

Hyperkeratotic lesion showing chevron like appearance of keratin

Fig. 8.4: 4X

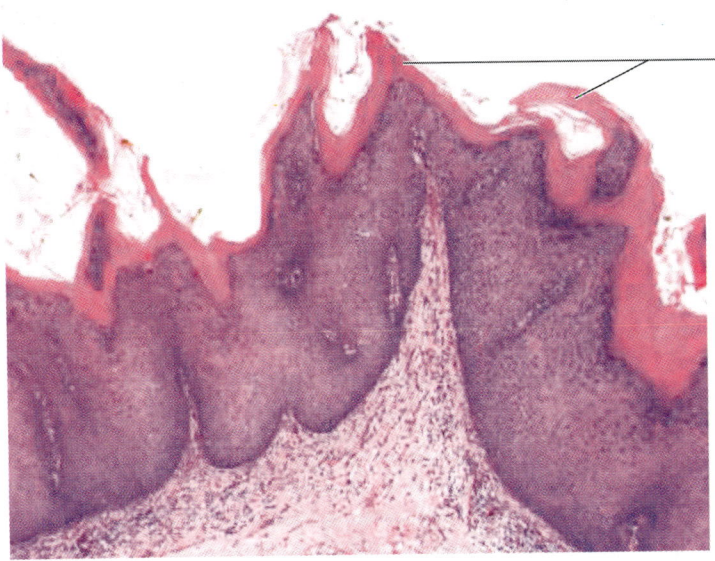

Hyperkeratotic lesions showing chevron appearance of keratin

Fig. 8.5: 10X

Key Points

- Parakeratin chevron (inverted V or eosinophilic spikes toward the surface) can be seen as pointed projections above or within superficial epithelial cells.
- Chevron (etymology): French word for rafters or shallow roof.
- Chevron (definition): Resembling a figure, pattern or object having a shape of a V or an inverted V.

ORAL LICHEN PLANUS (OLP)

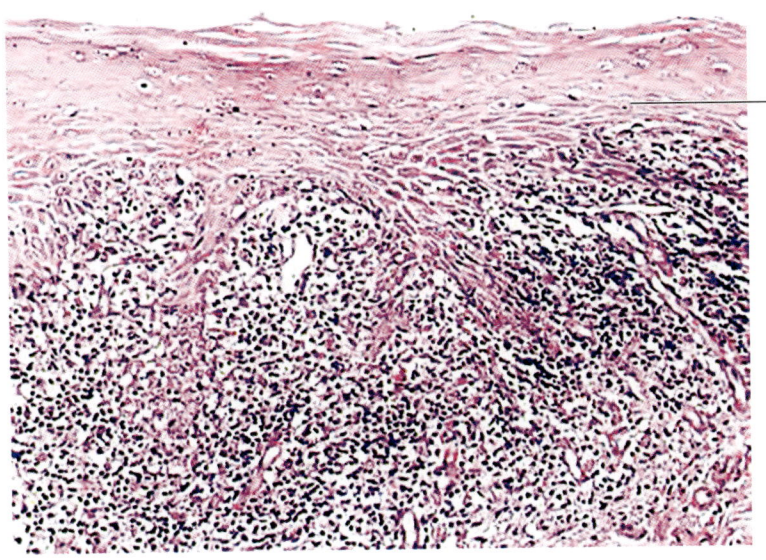

Hyperkeratotic lesion with subepithelial band of chronic inflammatory cell infiltrate

Fig. 8.6: 4X

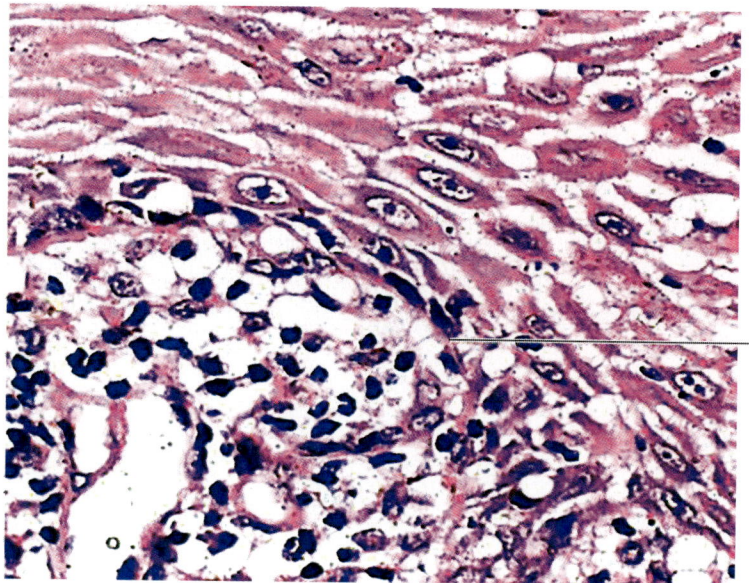

Liquefactive degeneration of basal cell and basement membrane

Fig. 8.7: 40X

Key Points

- Oral lichen planus (OLP) is a mucocutaneous multifactorial disease affecting the skin and mucosa, first described in 1869 by Erasmus Wilson.
- OLP affects 1–2% of the general population whereas, prevalence of cutaneous lichen planus (CLP) is estimated to be <1% of the population.
- The mean age is fifth decade, with slight female predilection and most common site affected is posterior buccal mucosa followed by tongue, gingiva and lower lip.
- OLP has been associated with multiple etiological factors like autoimmunity, anxiety, genetic predisposition, contact allergens in dental restorative materials or toothpastes, drug reactions, mechanical trauma, systemic conditions, bacterial, viral, fungal infections and tobacco habits.
- The association between OLP and viral infections, such as herpes simplex virus, Epstein—Barr virus, human papilloma virus, hepatitis B virus (HBV) and hepatitis C virus (HCV) have been reported.
- The most extensively studied virus is HCV, but its association with OLP remains controversial.

Histopathological Picture

OLP microscopically is characterized by a combination of features, such as:
- Orthokeratosis or parakeratosis.
- Acanthosis or atrophy of the epithelium.
- Basal cell degeneration.
- Loss of rete-ridges or saw tooth rete-ridges.
- Presence of Civatte bodies (apoptotic keratinocyte).
- Subepithelial band of predominantly lymphocytic infiltration, in the upper lamina propria and at times melanin incontinence.

Additional Point

In the past oral lichen planus was considered as an oral potentially malignant disorder. However, a recent evidence suggests that it is an oral lichenoid lesion/reaction which shows premalignant behavior.

ORAL SUBMUCOUS FIBROSIS (OSMF)

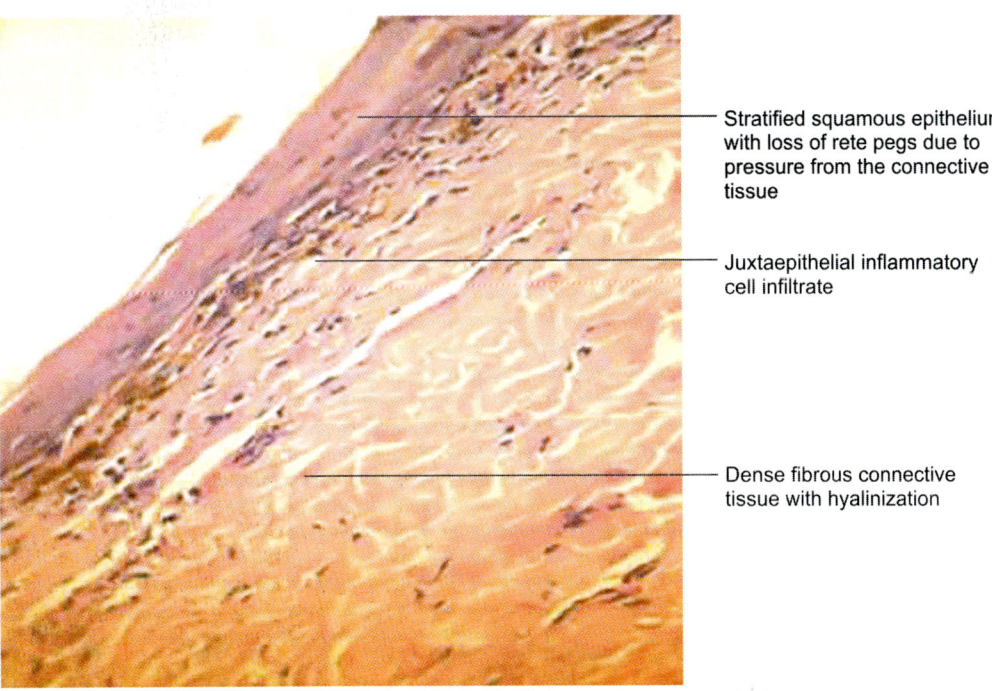

Stratified squamous epithelium with loss of rete pegs due to pressure from the connective tissue

Juxtaepithelial inflammatory cell infiltrate

Dense fibrous connective tissue with hyalinization

Fig. 8.8: 10X

Key Points

- Pindborg in 1966 defined OSMF as 'a chronic insidious disease affecting any part of oral cavity and sometimes the pharynx. Although occasionally preceded by and/or associated with vesicle formation, it is always associated with a juxtaepithelial inflammatory reaction followed by a fibroelastic change of lamina propria, with epithelial atrophy leading to stiffness of oral mucosa causing trismus and inability to eat'.
- OSMF occurs at any age but is most commonly seen in adolescents and adults especially between 16 and 35 years.
- It is predominantly seen in Southeast Asia and Indian subcontinent with few cases reported from South Africa, Greece and United Kingdom.
- The etiology of OSMF is multifactorial but areca nut chewing is the main causative agent. The possible etiological factors often discussed are:
  a. Areca nut (alkaoid)
  b. Capsaicin in chillies
  c. Micronutrient deficiencies of iron, zinc
  d. Vitamins deficiencies.

- The reasons for the rapid increase in the prevalence is due to an upsurge in the popularity of commercially prepared areca nut and tobacco preparations—gutkha, pan masala, mawa, flavored supari, etc.
- Burning sensation of mouth (stomatopyrosis) and formation of vesicles.
- Ulceration or recurrent stomatitis with excessive salivation or xerostomia and defective gustatory sensations.
- Stiffening of certain areas of oral mucosa with difficulty in opening mouth and swallowing.

Histopathological Picture

Epithelial Changes

- The epithelial changes in the different stages of OSMF are predominantly hyperplasia (early) and atrophy (advanced), associated with an increased tendency for keratinizing dysplasia.
- The atrophic epithelium also exhibits intracellular edema, signet cells and epithelial atypia (focal dysplasia).

Connective Tissue Changes

- Pindborg et al (1966) has described four consecutive stages in oral submucous fibrosis cases based on sections stained with hematoxylin and eosin:

  The changes are based on following criteria:
  a. Presence or absence of edema
  b. Nature of the collagen bundles
  c. Overall fibroblastic response
  d. State of the blood vessels
  e. Predominant cell type in the inflammatory exudates.
- **Early stage:** Fine fibrillar collagen dispersed with marked edema and strong fibroblastic response showing plump young fibroblasts containing abundant cytoplasm will be observed.
- The blood vessels are occasionally normal, but more often they are dilated and congested.
- Inflammatory cells, mainly polymorphonuclear leukocytes with occasional eosinophils, are present.
- As the lesion progress juxta-epithelial area shows early hyalinization.
- In the later stages, collagen is completely hyalinized and is seen as a smooth sheet with no distinct bundles or edema. The hyalinized connective tissue becomes hypocellular with thin elongated cells with vestigial nucleus at rare intervals along the bundles. Blood vessels are completely obliterated or narrowed.
- Melanin containing cells in the lamina propria are surrounded by dense collagen, which explains the clinically observed loss of pigmentation.

Additional Point

Susrutha in ancient medicine described a condition similar to OSMF as 'vidari'.

Chapter

9

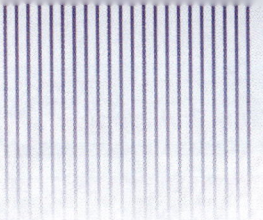

Epithelial Tumors

SQUAMOUS PAPILLOMA

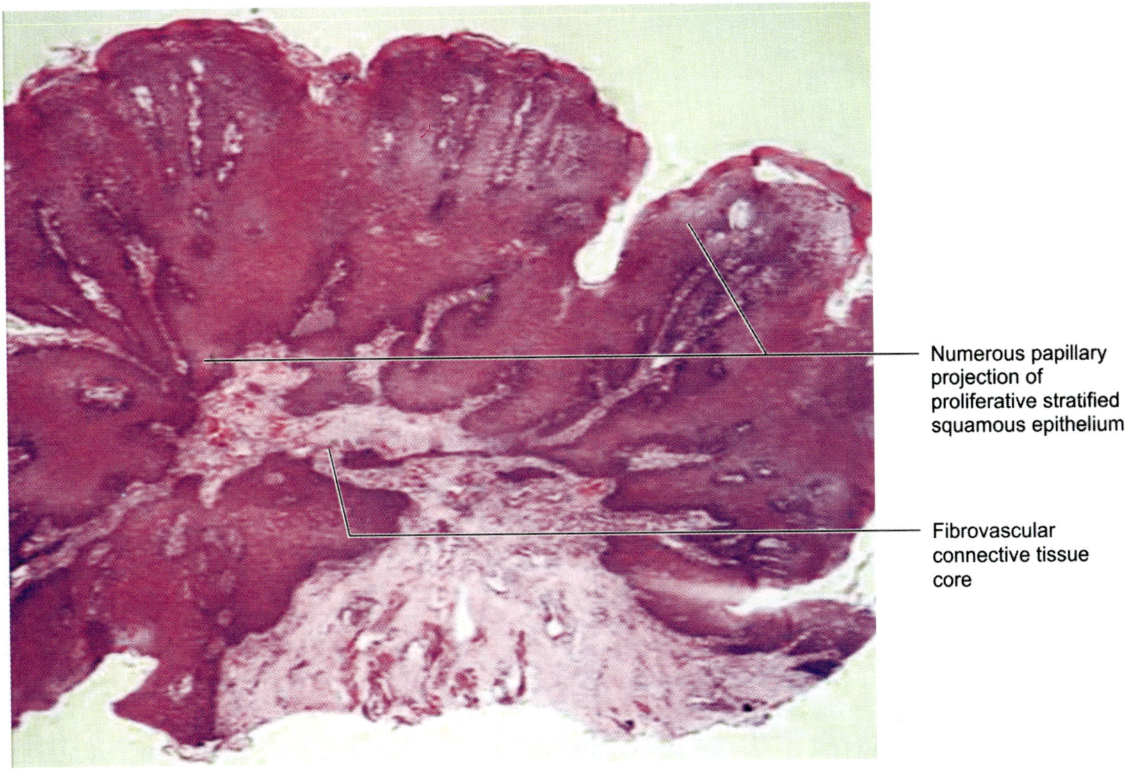

Numerous papillary projection of proliferative stratified squamous epithelium
Fibrovascular connective tissue core

Fig. 9.1: 10X

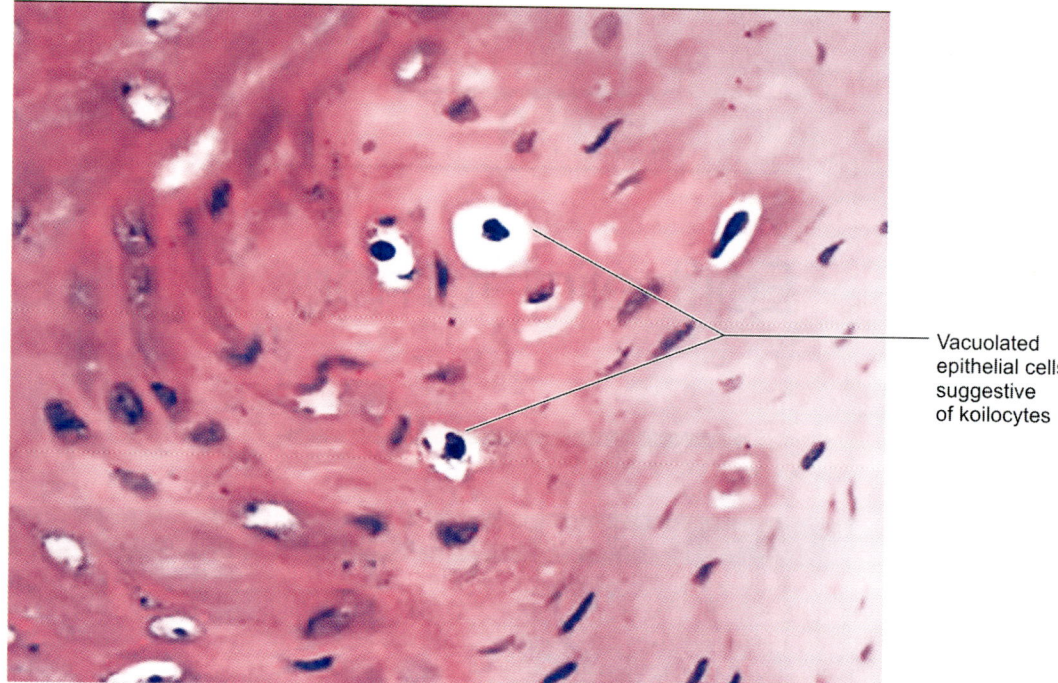

Vacuolated
epithelial cells
suggestive
of koilocytes

Fig. 9.2: 40X

Key Points
- Associated with human papilloma virus, HPV type 6 and 11.
- Occurs at any age.
- Intraorally most commonly found on the tongue, lips, buccal mucosa, gingiva and palate, particularly the area adjacent to the uvula.
- Exophytic growth made-up of numerous, small finger like projections which result in a lesion with a roughened, verrucous or 'cauliflower like' surface.
- It is nearly always a well-circumscribed pedunculated tumor, occasionally sessile.
- It is painless, usually white but sometimes pink in color.

Histopathological Picture
- The microscopic appearance of the papilloma is characteristic and consists of many long, thin, finger-like projections extending above the surface of the mucosa, each made-up of a continuous layer of stratified squamous epithelium and containing a thin, central connective tissue core which supports the nutrient blood vessels.
- Koilocytes (HPV altered epithelial cells with perinuclear clear spaces and nuclear pyknosis) may or may not be found in the superficial layers of the epithelium. Vacuolated epithelial cells suggestive of koilocytes.

ORAL SQUAMOUS CELL CARCINOMA (OSCC)

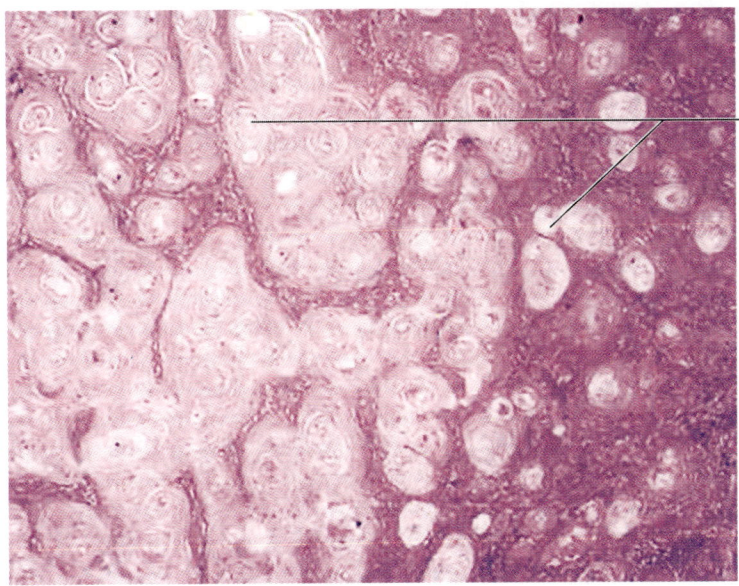

Lesional tissue consisting of numerous keratin pearls and malignant epithelial cells

Fig. 9.3: 4X

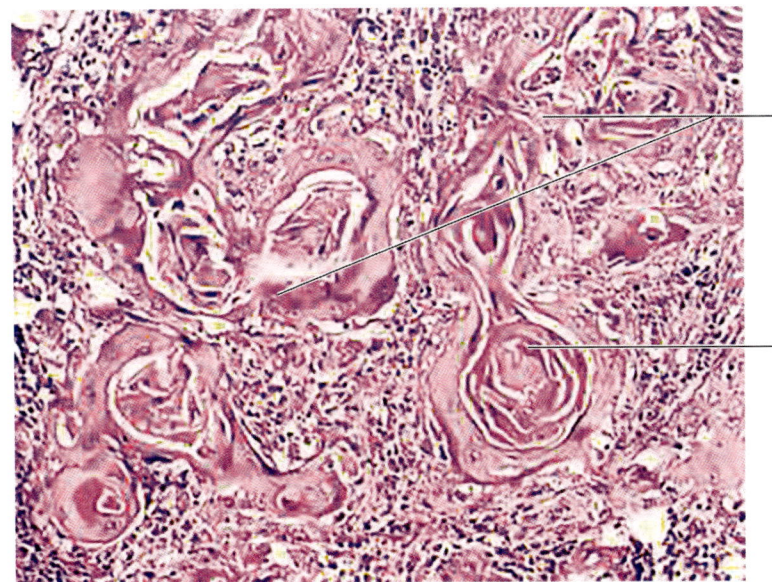

Connective tissue is infiltrated with malignant epithelial cells in the form of island, pearls and individual cells

Keratin pearl within the connective tissue

Fig. 9.4: 10X

Sarcomatoid Type OSCC (Poorly Differentiated Carcinoma)

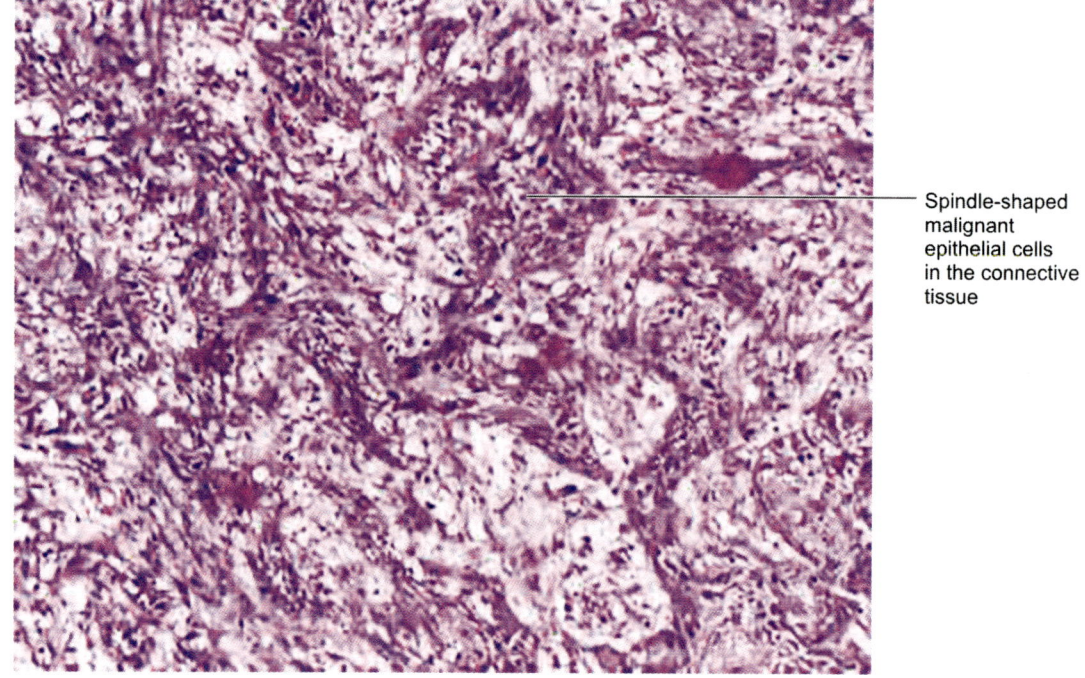

Spindle-shaped
malignant
epithelial cells
in the connective
tissue

Fig. 9.5: 10X

Key Points
- OSCC and its variants constitute over 90% of the oral malignancies.
- According to the data extracted from Globocan 2012, in India the overall oral cancer ranks third amongst all types of cancer, in terms of incidence and mortality and first among the males and fifth among the females.
- Oral squamous cell carcinoma is described as an invasive epithelial neoplasm with varying degrees of squamous differentiation having a propensity to early and extensive lymph node metastases.
- Occurs predominantly in alcohol and tobacco users.
- Generally seen in the 5th and 6th decade of life.
- Can involve any part of oral cavity depending upon the tobacco habit.
- In India alveobuccal complex is the most common site involved.
- Clinically, it is usually present as ulceroproliferative lesion.

Histopathological Picture
- In OSCC epithelium shows dysplastic changes and break in basement membrane.
- Malignant epithelial cells seen within connective tissue showing varying degree of differentiation.

- Histopathologic presentation can vary from well-differentiated to moderately to poorly differentiated type OSCC.
- In well-differentiated OSCC malignant epithelial cells show marked differentiation and closely resemble tissue of origin, i.e. epithelial cells. Numerous keratin pearl and epithelial pearl seen within connective tissue.
- In contrast, poorly differentiated tumors show marked cellular and nuclear alterations with little or no resemblance to squamous epithelium or those that lack keratin production.

Additional Points

- Treatment includes surgical excision and radiotherapy.
- Depending upon the clinical staging, histopathological grading the prognosis varies.
- Among the Indian population, the overall 5-year survival rate observed was 59.1% for localized cancer, 15.7% for cancers with regional extension and 1.6% for those with distant metastasis.

VERRUCOUS CARCINOMA

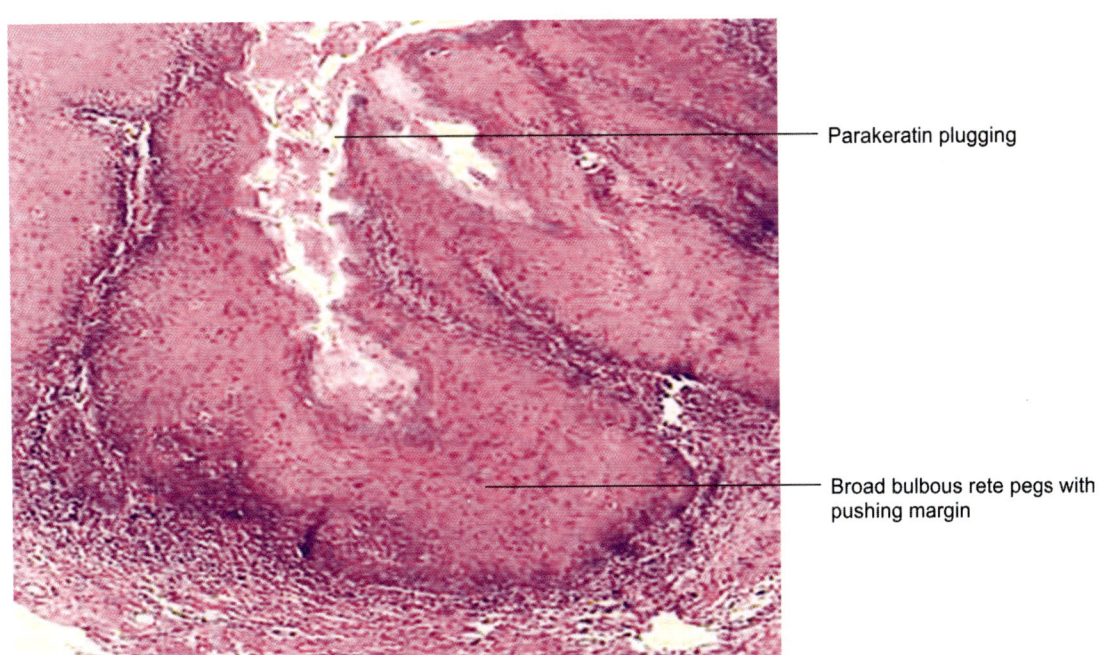

Parakeratin plugging

Broad bulbous rete pegs with pushing margin

Fig. 9.6: 4X

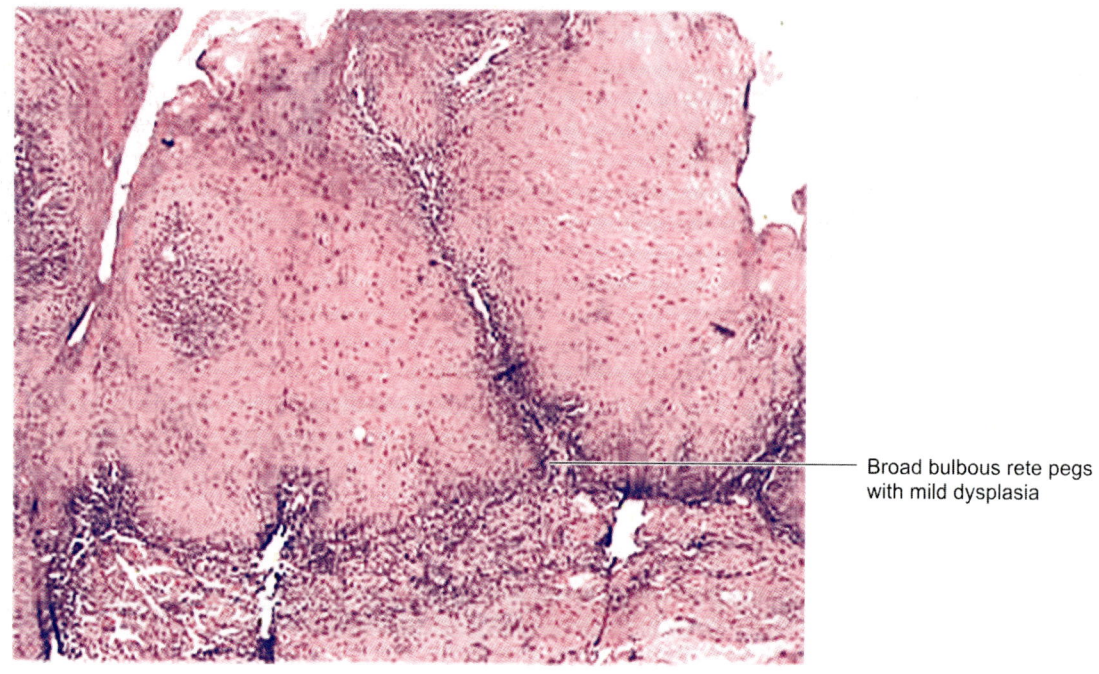

Broad bulbous rete pegs with mild dysplasia

Fig. 9.7: 10X

Key Points

- A warty variant of squamous cell carcinoma characterized by a predominantly exophytic overgrowth of well-differentiated keratinizing epithelium having minimal atypia and with locally destructive pushing margins at its interface with underlying connective tissue.
- Verrucous carcinoma is generally seen in elderly patients, the mean age of occurrence being 60–70 years, with nearly 75% of the lesions developing in males.
- Usually seen with tobacco chewing or snuff habit.
- There may be a significant endophytic component and the invading margin is usually below the level of the surrounding mucosa.
- The term verrucous hyperplasia describes an exophytic overgrowth of well-differentiated keratinizing epithelium that is similar to verrucous carcinoma but without the destructive pushing border at its interface with the underlying connective tissue.
- The vast majority of cases occur on the buccal mucosa and gingiva or alveolar ridge.
- The neoplasm is chiefly exophytic and appears papillary in nature, with a pebbly surface which is sometimes covered by a white leukoplakic film.
- Regional lymph nodes are often tender and enlarged, simulating metastatic tumor, but this node involvement is usually inflammatory.

Histopathological Picture

- Verrucous carcinoma histopathologically shows marked epithelial proliferation with down growth of epithelium into the connective tissue but usually without a pattern of true invasion.
- The epithelium is well-differentiated and shows little mitotic activity, little or no cytological atypia, pleomorphism or hyperchromatism.
- Parakeratin plugging also occurs extending into the epithelium. The parakeratin lining the clefts with the parakeratin plugging is the hallmark of verrucous carcinoma.

Additional Points

- Also called snuff dipper's cancer, Ackerman's tumor.
- Difficulty in diagnosis can occur due to extremely thick layers of keratin and hyperplastic epithelium leading to insufficient depth of biopsy, to include underlying connective tissue.
- Always rule out the possibility of oral squamous cell carcinoma in case of verrucous carcinoma.

Dental Caries

PIT AND FISSURE CARIES

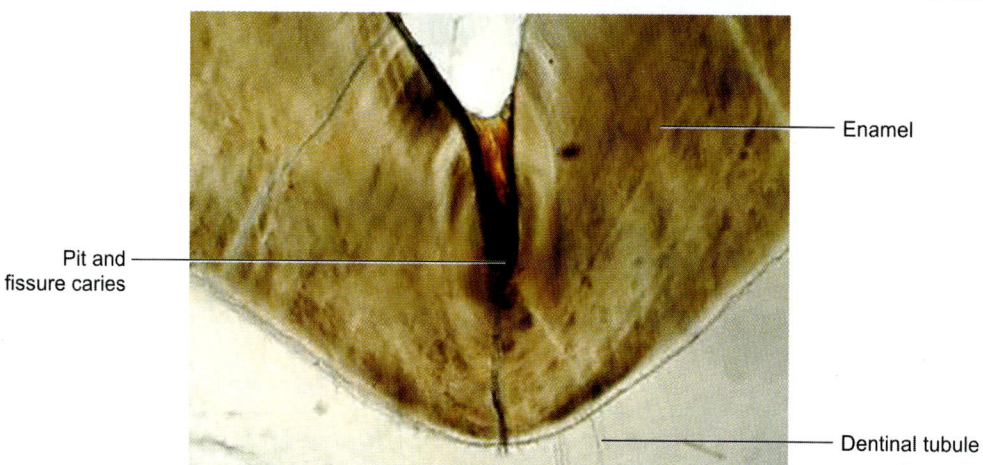

Enamel

Pit and
fissure caries

Dentinal tubule

Fig. 10.1: 4X

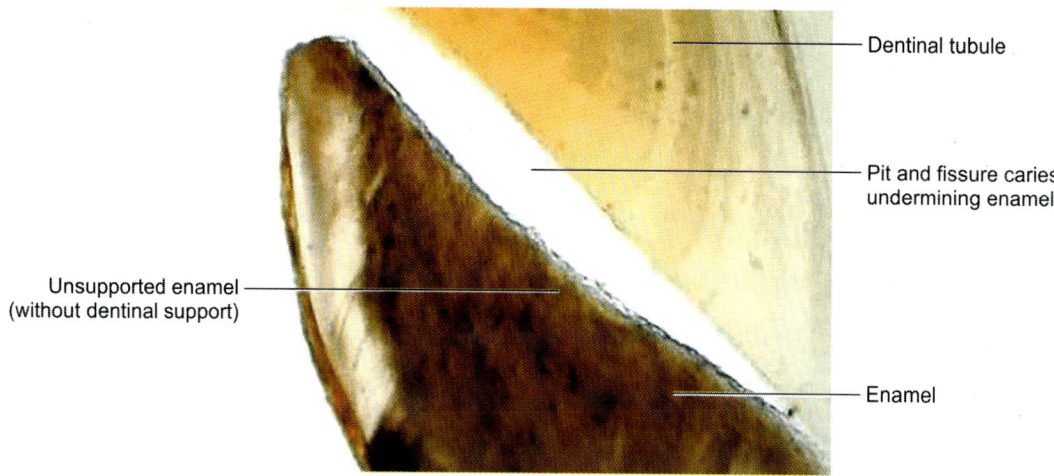

Dentinal tubule

Pit and fissure caries
undermining enamel

Unsupported enamel
(without dentinal support)

Enamel

Fig. 10.2: 4X

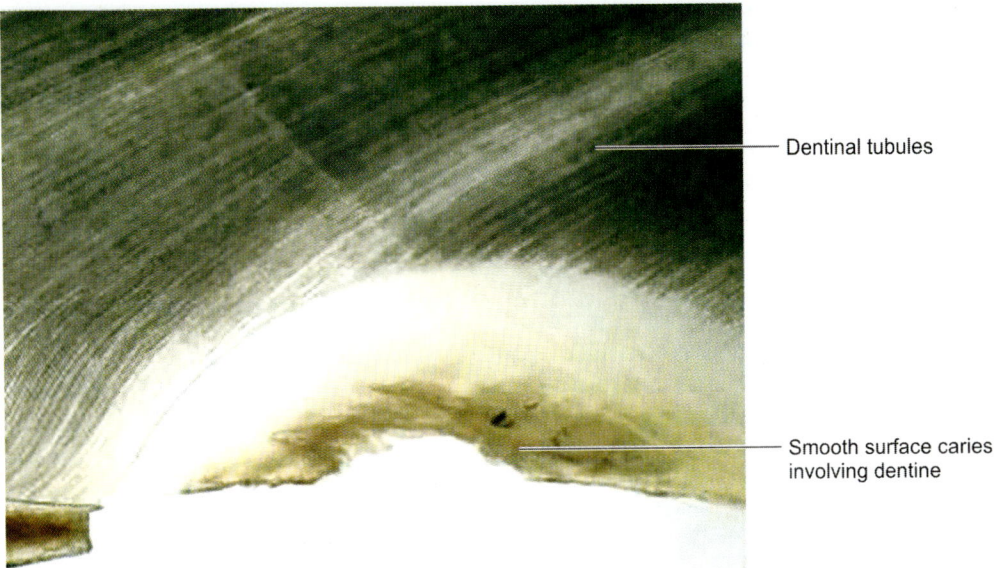

Dentinal tubules

Smooth surface caries
involving dentine

Fig. 10.3: 4X

Key Points

- Dental caries is an irreversible polymicrobial disease of the calcified tissues of the teeth.
- It has multifactorial etiology.
- Deep and narrow pits and fissures are more prone to caries then shallow and wide pit and fissures.
- The word caries is derived from the Latin word meaning 'rot' or 'decay'.
- At a critical pH of 5.5, the tooth minerals act as buffers and they loose calcium and phosphate ions into the plaque.
- Most common organism associated with pit and fissure caries is streptococcus mutans.
- After reaching dentinoenamel junction (DEJ), caries spread rapidly and laterally into the dentin along the dentinal tubules leading to unsupported enamel.
- General shape of pit an fissure lesion is triangular or cone-shaped with its apex at the outer surface and base toward the dentinoenamel junction, opposite of that occurrs on smooth surface.
- Early microscopic change in enamel caries is loss of the interprismatic or interrod substance of the enamel with increased prominence of the rods or accentuation of the incremental lines of Retzius.
- Primary smooth surface caries develops on the proximal surfaces of the teeth or on the cervical third of the buccal and lingual surfaces.

DENTINAL CARIES

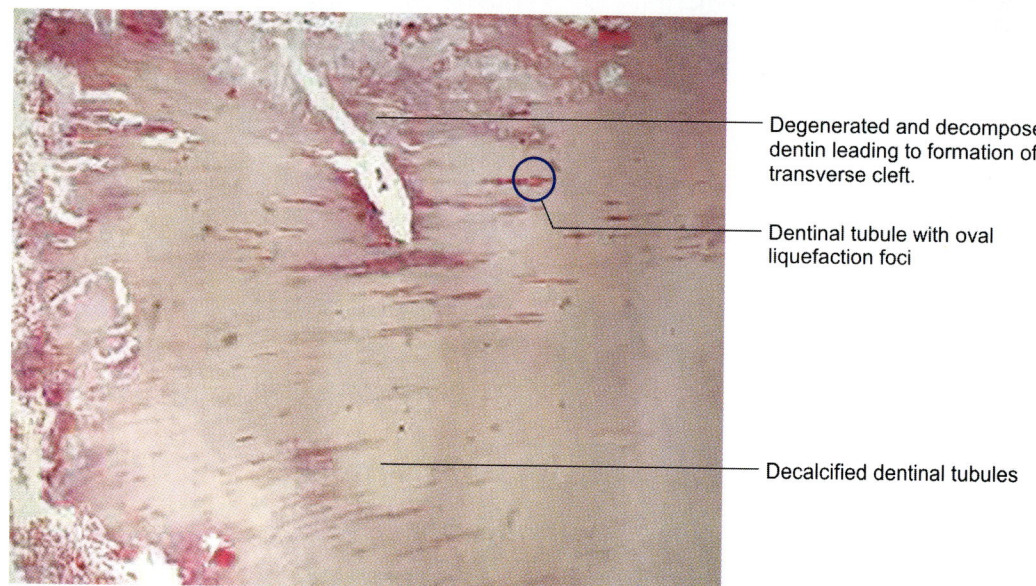

Degenerated and decomposed dentin leading to formation of transverse cleft.

Dentinal tubule with oval liquefaction foci

Decalcified dentinal tubules

Fig. 10.4: 10X

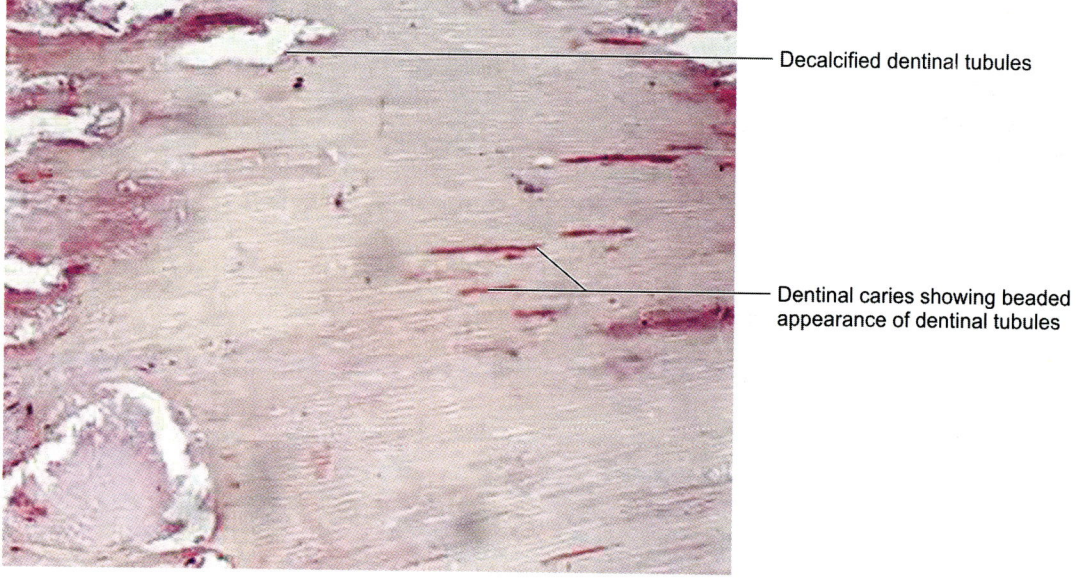

Decalcified dentinal tubules

Dentinal caries showing beaded appearance of dentinal tubules

Fig. 10.5: 10X

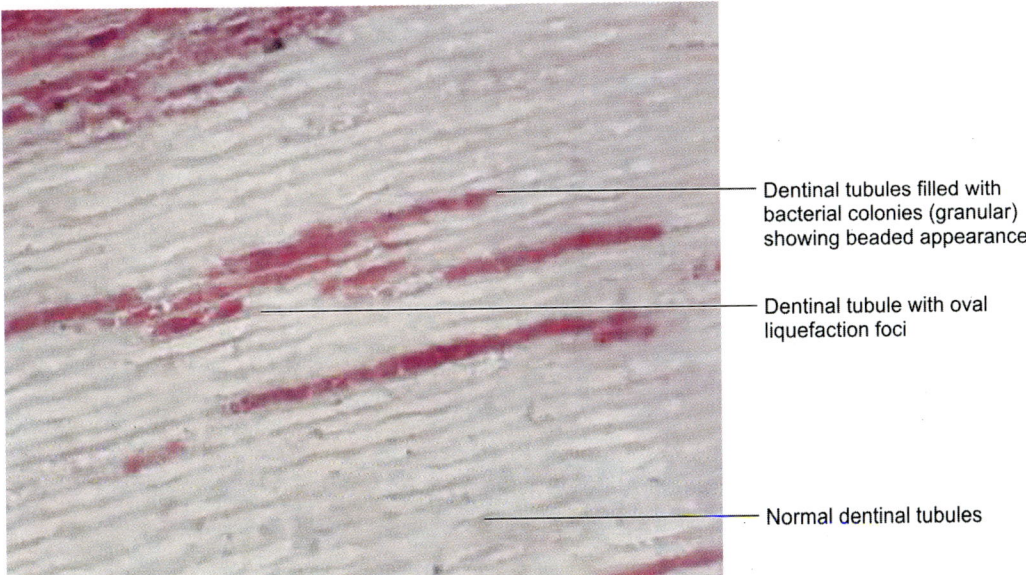

Dentinal tubules filled with bacterial colonies (granular) showing beaded appearance

Dentinal tubule with oval liquefaction foci

Normal dentinal tubules

Fig. 10.6: 40X

Histopathological Picture

- Due to penetration and colonization of bacteria in the dentinal tubules there is beaded appearance, which ultimately leads to formation of varicosities caused by bacterial degradation.
- With development of more varicosities in adjacent area, coalescing occurs leading to oval liquefaction foci.
- They are called liquefaction foci because they are filled with fluid and often flatten and distort adjacent tubules by exerting pressure.
- Later on transverse clefts are formed due to dentin disintegration which runs at right angles to tubules.

Chapter

11

Pulpal Pathologies

PULPITIS

Acute Pulpitis

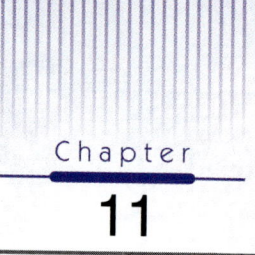

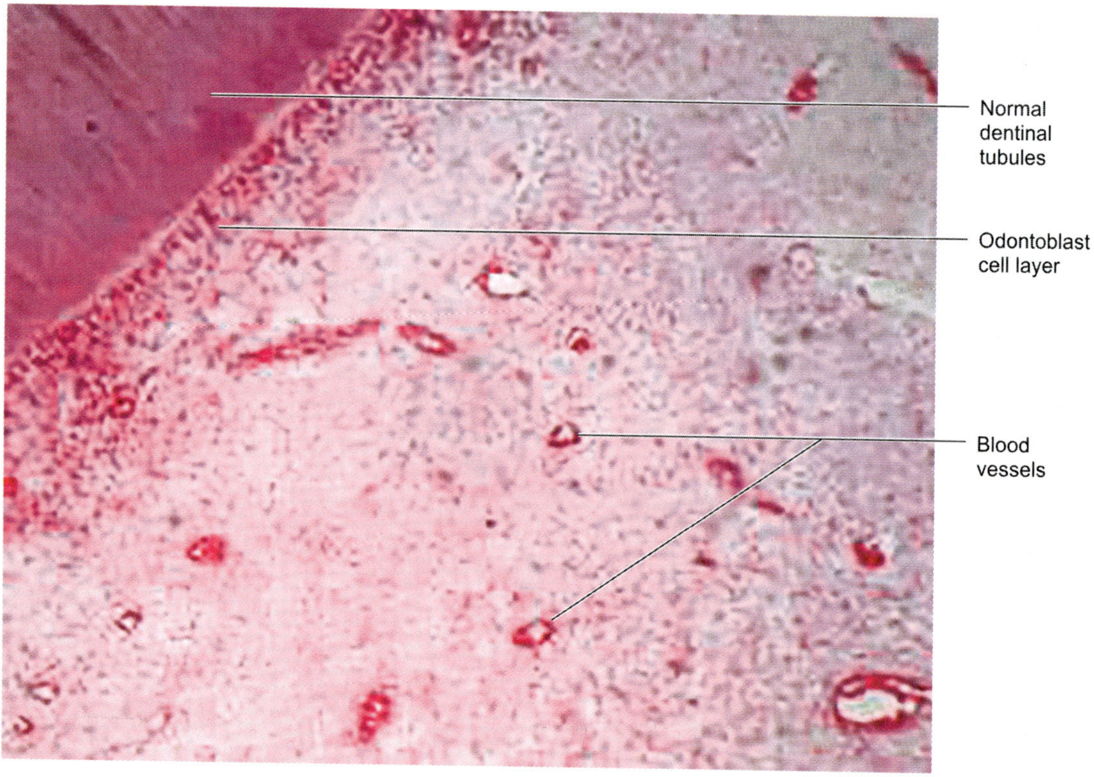

Normal dentinal tubules
Odontoblast cell layer
Blood vessels

Fig. 11.1: 4X

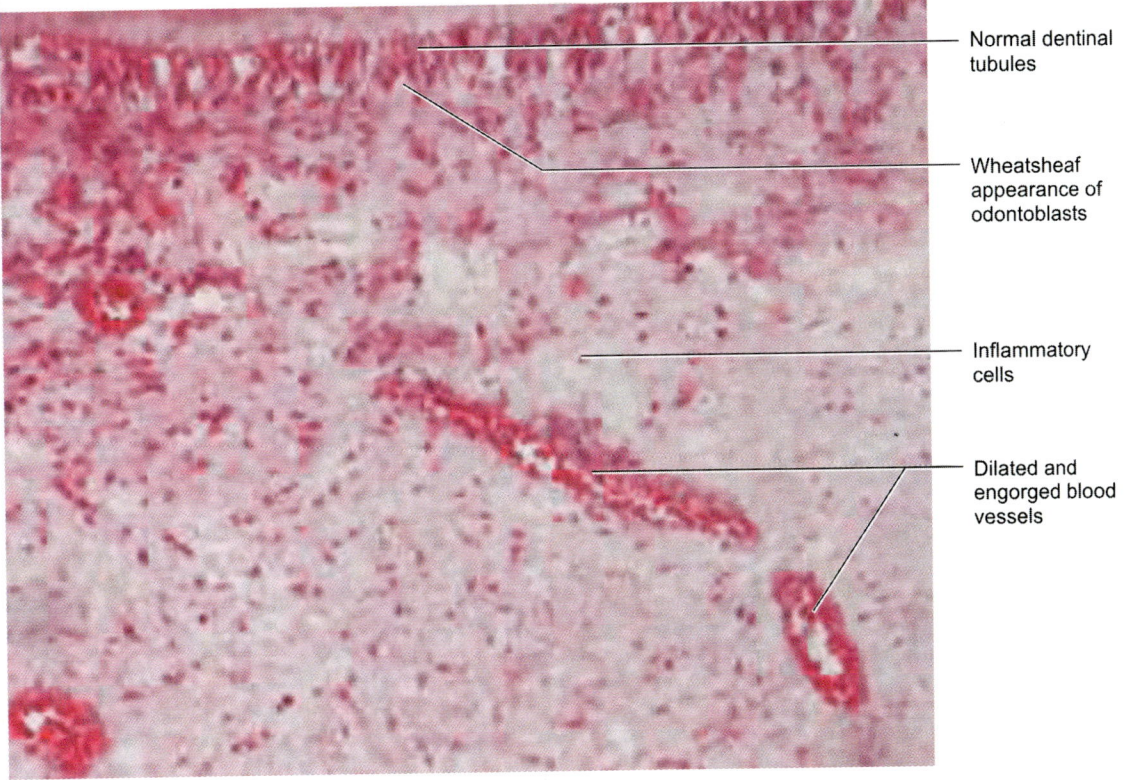

Normal dentinal tubules

Wheatsheaf appearance of odontoblasts

Inflammatory cells

Dilated and engorged blood vessels

Fig. 11.2: 4X

Histopathological Picture

- Vascular dilatation accompanied by the accumulation of edema fluid in the connective tissue.
- Inflammatory cell infiltrate chiefly in the form of neutrophils.
- Initially focal areas of polymorphonuclear leukocytes are seen and the rest of the pulpal tissue appears relatively normal.
- With passage of time pressure in the pulp increase due to inflammatory exudate leading to local collapse of circulation resulting in hypoxia and anoxia. Which ultimately leads to localized destruction and the formation of abscess, known as a pulp abscess.

ACUTE PULPITIS WITH ABSCESS

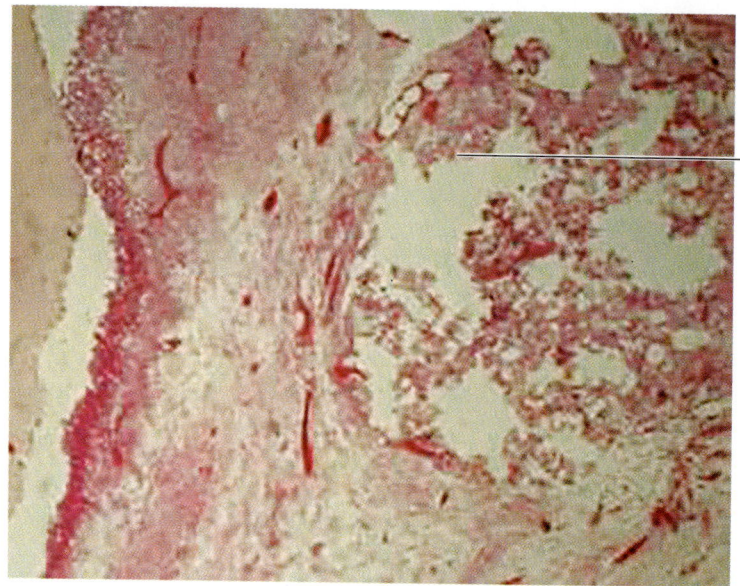

Pulp tissue with empty spaces and degenerated cells (abscess)

Fig. 11.3: 4X

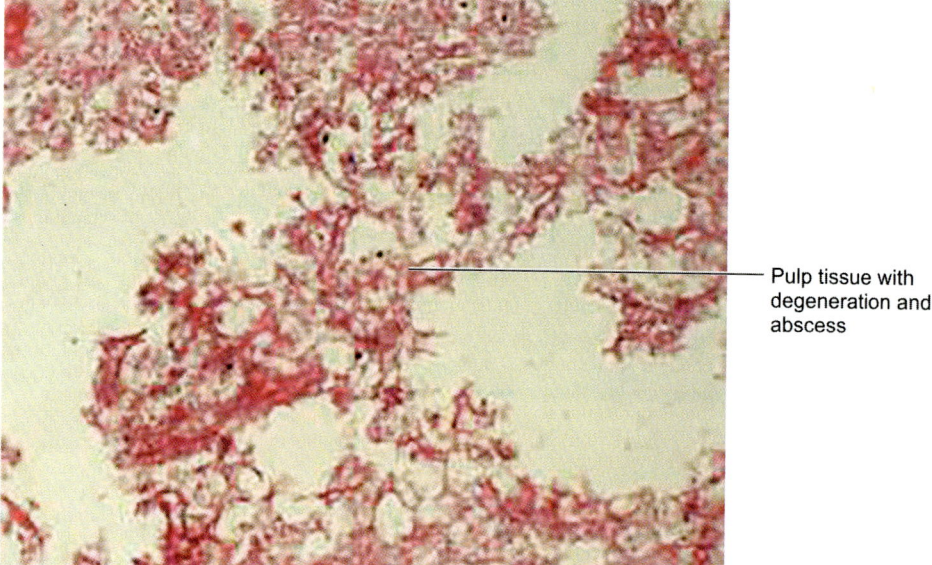

Pulp tissue with degeneration and abscess

Fig. 11.4: 10X

Histopathological Picture

- Histopathological picture is similar to acute pulpitis with abcess formation.
- Odontoblast shows wheatsheafing effect. Hydropic degeneration in odontoblast.

CHRONIC PULPITIS

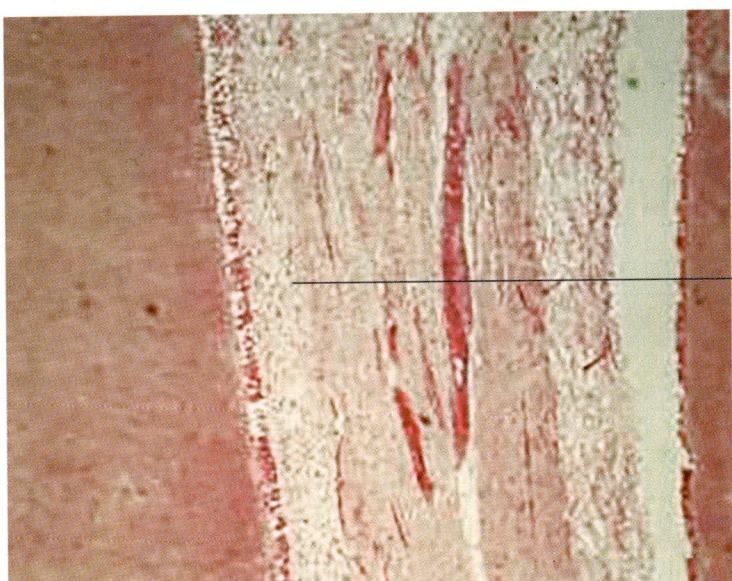

Pulp tissue with chronic inflammatory cell infiltrate

Fig. 11.5: 4X

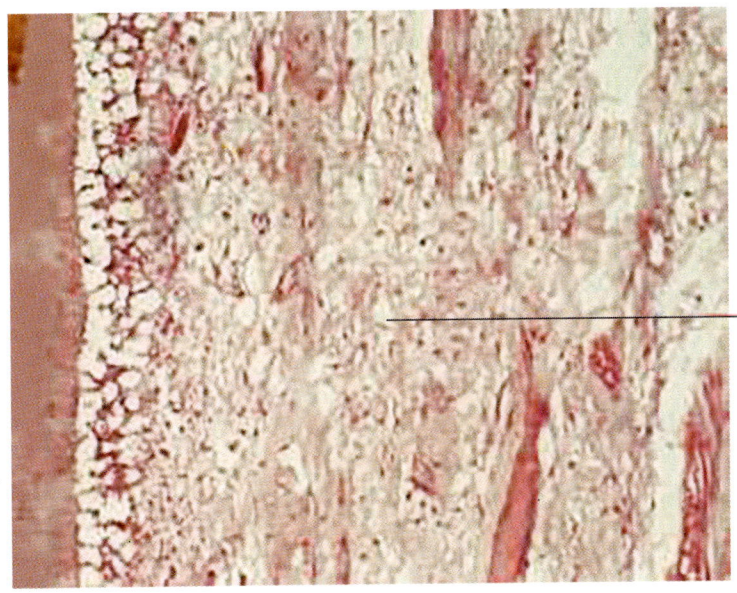

Pulp tissue with chronic inflammatory cell infiltrate and reactive fibrosis

Fig. 11.6: 10X

CHRONIC PULPITIS WITH ABSCESS

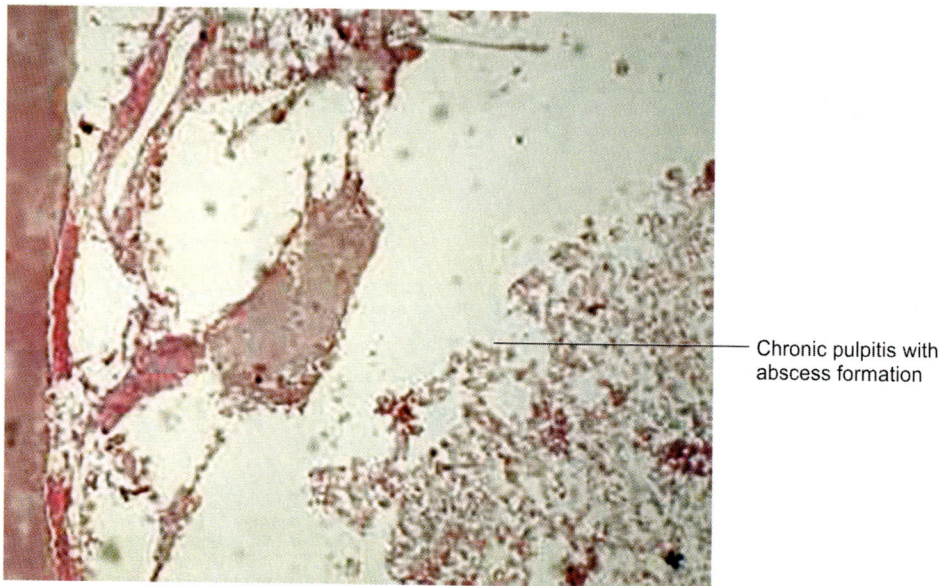

Chronic pulpitis with abscess formation

Fig. 11.7: 10X

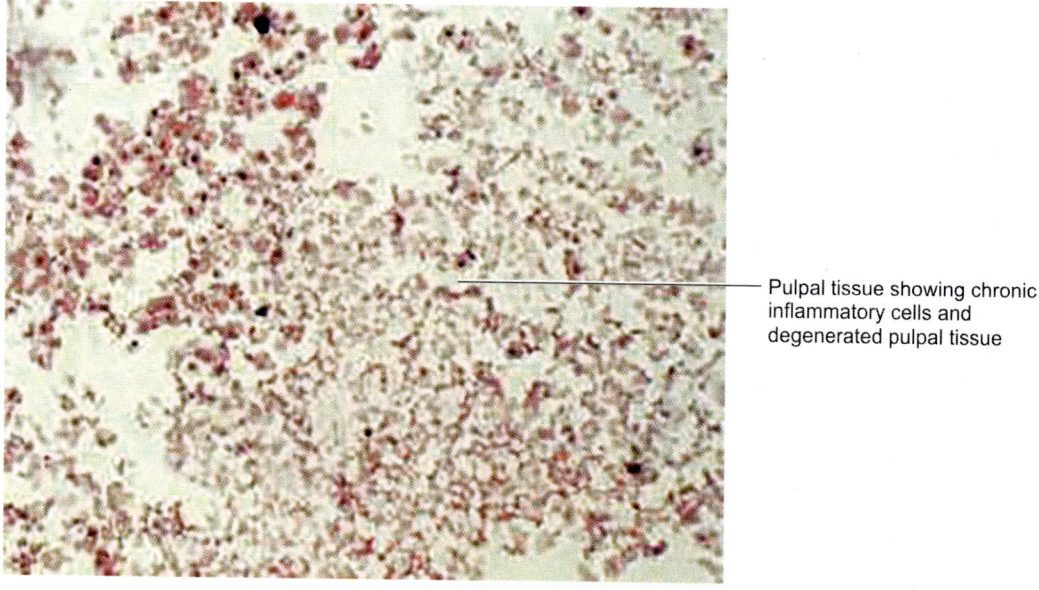

Pulpal tissue showing chronic inflammatory cells and degenerated pulpal tissue

Fig. 11.8: 10X

PULP FIBROSIS

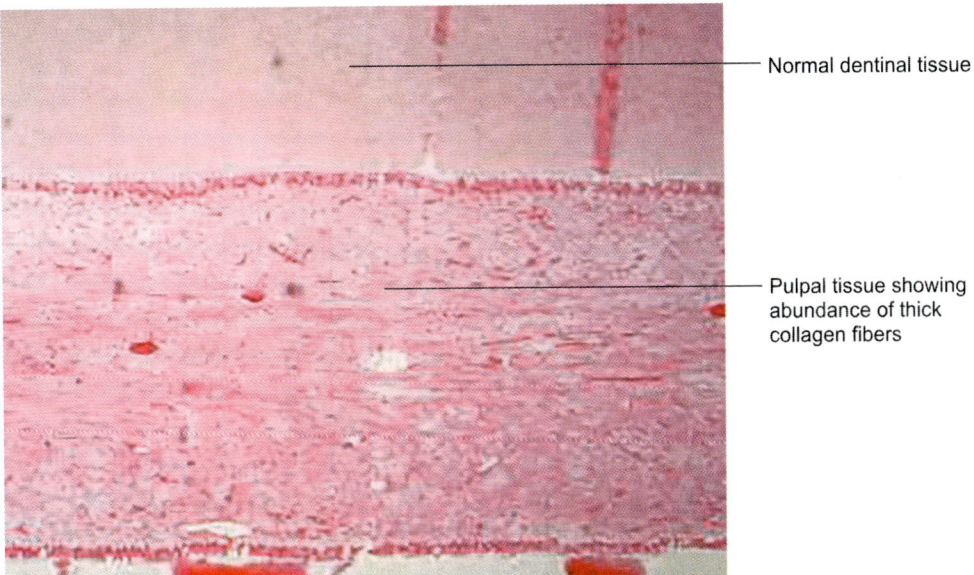

Normal dentinal tissue

Pulpal tissue showing abundance of thick collagen fibers

Fig. 11.9: 4X

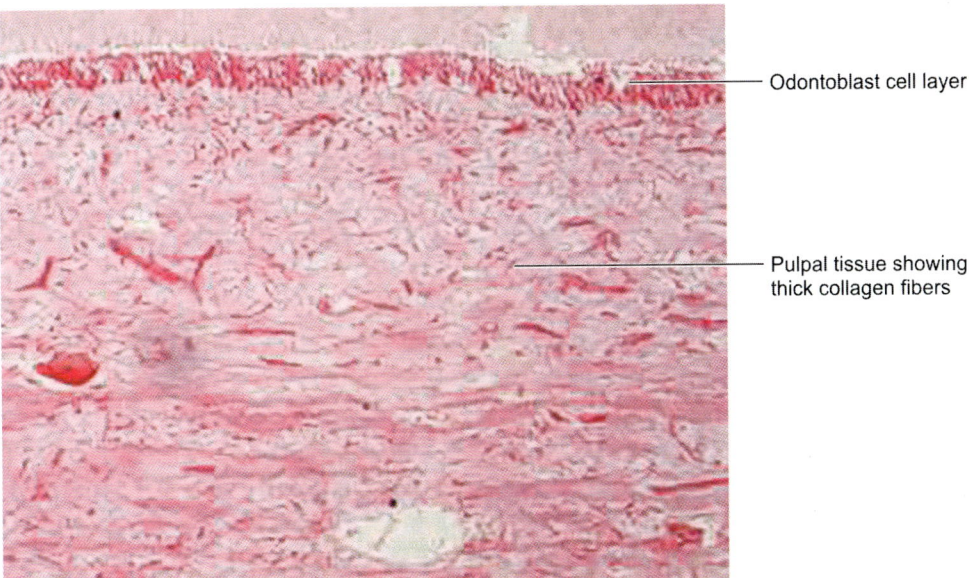

Odontoblast cell layer

Pulpal tissue showing thick collagen fibers

Fig. 11.10: 10X

Key Points

- Pulp fibrosis is an aging phenomenon.
- Pulp is a loose connective tissue.
- With aging or insult to external factors fibers in the pulp becomes thick leading to pulp fibrosis.
- Over a period of time pulp fibrosis may lead to calcification which may be diffuse or as a denticle.

PULP CALCIFICATION

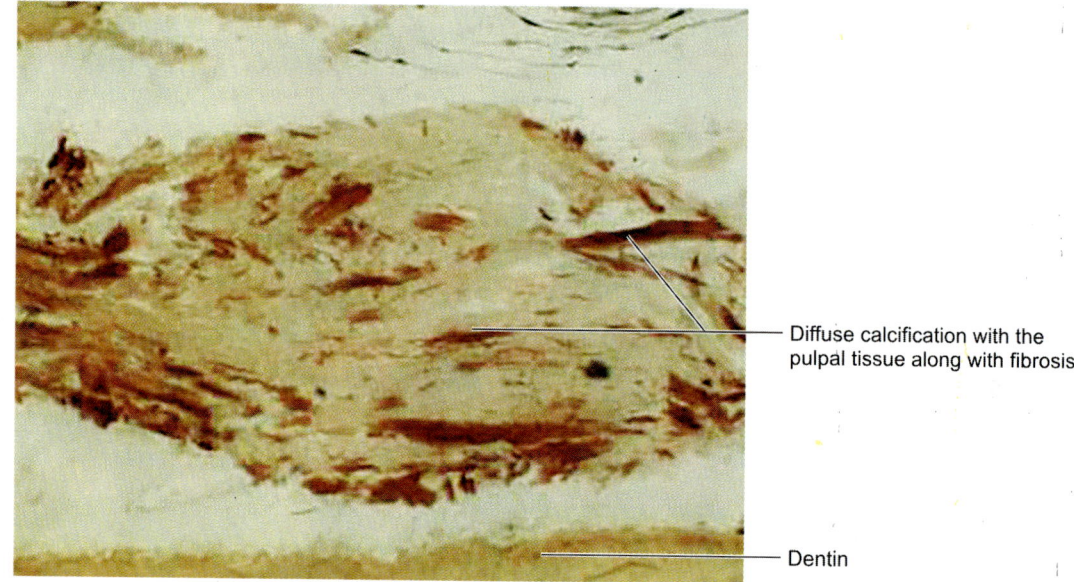

Diffuse calcification with the pulpal tissue along with fibrosis

Dentin

Fig. 11.11: 10X

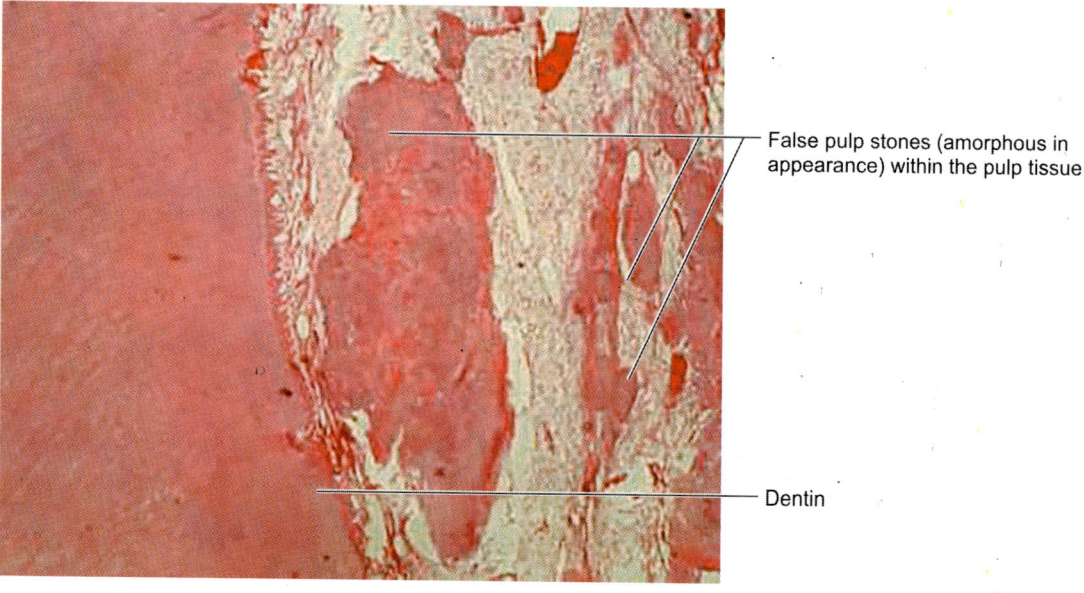

False pulp stones (amorphous in appearance) within the pulp tissue

Dentin

Fig. 11.12a: 10X

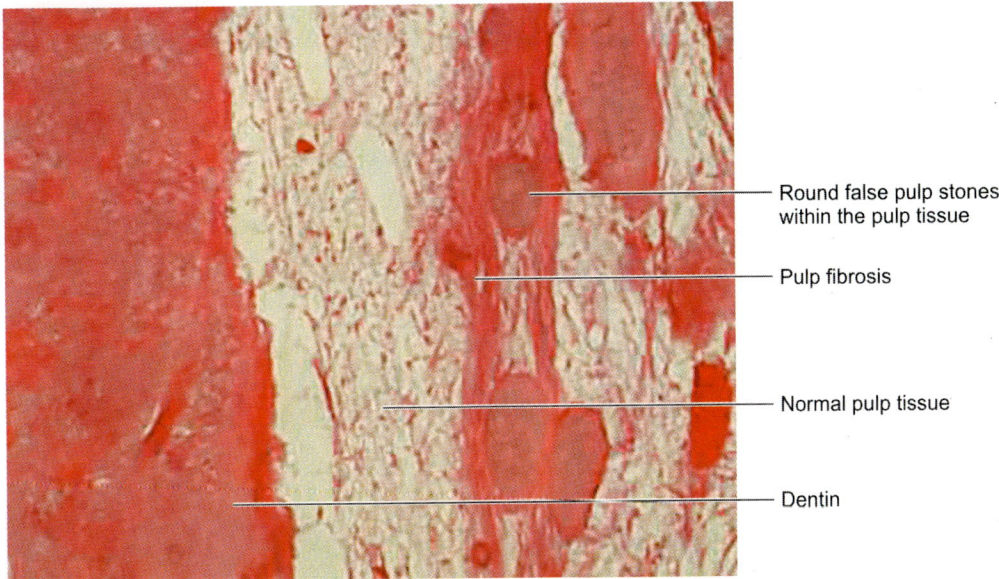

Round false pulp stones within the pulp tissue

Pulp fibrosis

Normal pulp tissue

Dentin

Fig. 11.12b: 10X

Key Points

- Hard tissue formation in pulp is aging phenomenon.
- Hard tissue can be seen as diffuse calcification and/or pulp stone (denticle).
- Denticles are mostly seen in the pulp chamber than in the root canal.
- Diffuse calcification is predominately seen in the root canals of teeth.
- Also termed calcific degeneration.
- Diffuse calcification usually appear as amorphous, unorganized linear strands or columns mostly around the blood vessels and nerve tissue.
- With increase in fibrous content of pulp chances of calcification increases, as thick collagen fibers act as nidus for mineral deposition.

Additional Point

Calcification within the pulp lead to difficulty in root canal treatment.

PULP NECROSIS

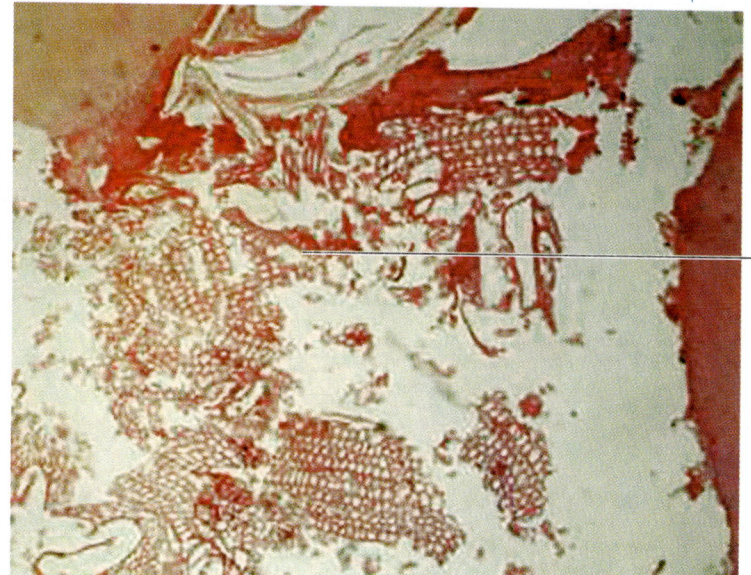

Pulpal tissue showing degeneration and necrotic areas

Fig. 11.13a: 4X

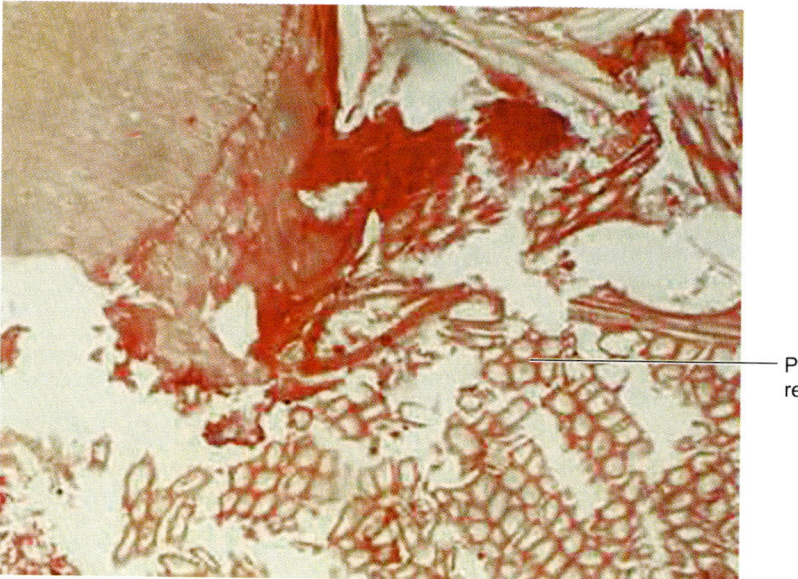

Pulpal tissue showing reticular degeneration

Fig. 11.13b: 4X

Histopathological Picture

- With passage of time as duration of pulpitis increases, pressure within the pulp chamber increase due to inflammatory exudate leading to local collapse of circulation resulting in hypoxia and anoxia which ultimately leads to necrosis of pulpal tissue.
- Sometimes the pattern of degeneration is in the form of network called reticular degeneration.

PULP POLYP

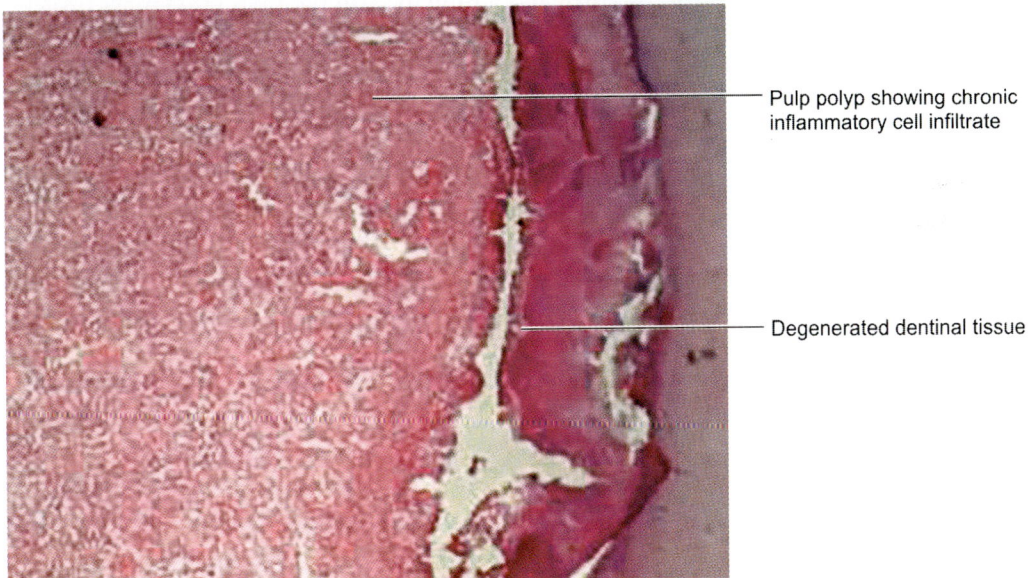

Pulp polyp showing chronic inflammatory cell infiltrate

Degenerated dentinal tissue

Fig. 11.14: 4X

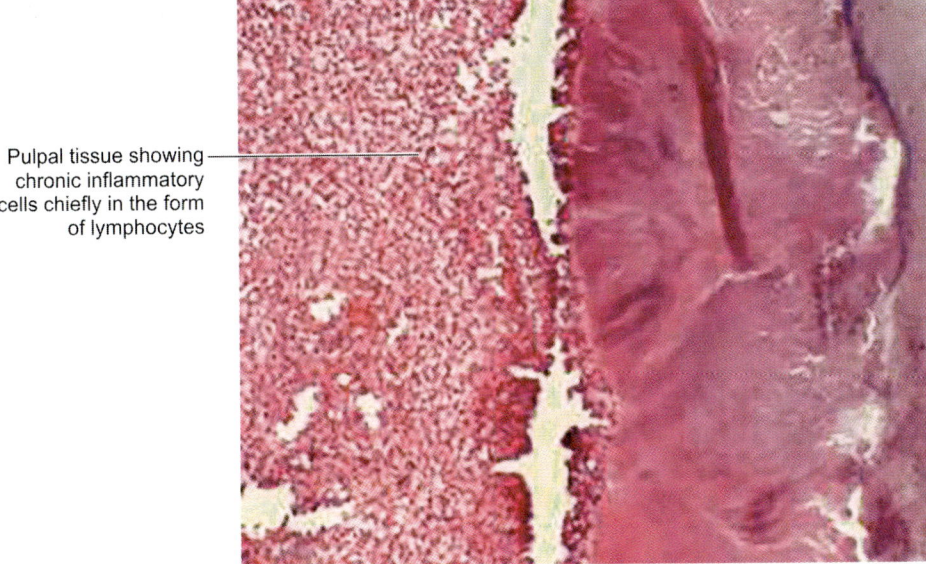

Pulpal tissue showing chronic inflammatory cells chiefly in the form of lymphocytes

Fig. 11.15: 4X

Key Points

- Unique form of pulpitis wherein the inflamed pulp, instead of suppuration reacts by excessive and exuberant proliferation.
- Occurs either as a chronic lesion from the onset or acute pulpitis changing into chronic one.

- Seen exclusively in children and young adults.
- Involves teeth with large, open carious lesions.
- Granulation tissue grows out of the coronal opening to form pedunculated mass protruding into the oral cavity, so-called polyp.
- Color varies from cherry red (granulation tissue) to opaque white (keratinization).
- Most commonly involved teeth are the deciduous molars and the first permanent molars (blood supply to pulp is correspondingly good).

Histopathological Picture

- Lesional tissue usually shows hyperplastic granulation tissue made-up of delicate connective tissue fibers interspersed with variable numbers of small capillaries.
- Inflammatory cell infiltration, chiefly lymphocytes and plasma cells, sometimes admixed with polymorphonuclear leukocytes, is common.
- Granulation tissue may become epithelized, but origin of epithelial cells is controversial. (Normal viable desquamated epithelial cells in the saliva, cells from buccal mucosa or gingiva.)

Question and Answer Bank

1. Define cyst.

Ans. Cyst is defined as a pathological cavity having fluid, semifluid or gaseous contents and which is not created by the accumulation of pus which may or may not be lined by epithelium.

2. Difference between true cyst and pseudocyst with examples.

Ans. Basic morphology of cyst is cystic lumen, lining epithelium and connective tissue wall. True cyst are those cyst which are lined by lining epithelium and cyst which lack the lining epithelium are called pseudocyst.

True cyst: Radicular cyst, OKC, dentigerous cyst, etc.

Pseudocyst: Traumatic bone cyst, aneurysmal bone cyst, mucous extravasation phenomenon.

3. Why odontogenic cysts are basically classified as developmental and inflammatory odontogenic cysts? Give examples.

Ans. Developmental odontogenic cyst are those cyst which arise from the odontogenic tooth apparatus without any stimulus and resemble them.

Examples: Dentigerous cyst, OKC, OOC and lateral periodontal cyst. Those odontogenic cyst in which inflammation plays an important role in their formation are called inflammatory odontogenic cyst.

Examples: Radicular cyst, residual cyst and paradental cyst.

4. Cystic fluid in case of dentigerous and OKC.

Ans. In case of dentigerous cyst the fluid is usually a thin, watery yellow fluid, occasionally blood tinged or straw colored, whereas in case of OKC depending upon the amount of keratinization the fluid varies from straw colored to cheesy white in appearance.

5. Why OKC has high recurrence potential?

Ans: The causes and factors responsible for recurrence of OKC are:

- Incomplete removal of cystic lining.
- Thin and friable nature of epithelial lining.
- Higher level of cell proliferative activity in the lining epithelium.
- Budding in the basal layer of the lining epithelium.
- Supraepithelial and subepithelial split of the epithelial lining.
- Development of new OKC from satellite cyst/daughter cyst/cell rests.

6. Syndrome associated with different types of cyst.

Ans. Bilateral and multiple dentigerous cysts are usually found in association with a number of syndromes including cleidocranial dysplasia and Maroteaux-Lamy syndrome.

Multiple OKCs are seen in association with nevoid basal cell carcinoma syndrome.

7. What are Rushton bodies?

Ans. Rushton bodies are hyaline, tiny curvilinear linear or arc-shaped bodies, generally associated with the lining epithelium, that appear amorphous in structure, eosinophilic in reaction and brittle in nature.

8. What are Russell bodies?

Ans. Russell bodies are eosinophilic, large, homogeneous immunoglobulin-containing inclusions usually found in plasma cells undergoing excessive synthesis of immunoglobulins.

9. Difference between OKC and OOC.

Ans. • OOC is more aggressive than OKC.
 • OOC histopathologically shows orthokeratinization and OKC shows parakeratinization.
 • OOC shows prominent stratum granulosum.
 • In OOC the basal cell layer is cuboidal to flat.
 • OOC does not show any association with nevoid basal cell carcinoma syndrome.

10. What are various sources of origin for development of odontogenic cyst?

Ans. Various sources for development of odontogenic cysts are:
 • Rest of Serres
 • Rests of Malassez
 • Reduced enamel epithelium
 • Surface epithelium (peripheral type)
 • Odontogenic rest along the gubernacular dentis.

11. Different pathogenesis of radicular cyst.

Ans. 1. Stimulus from inflammation may lead to proliferation of rests of Malassez.
 2. Periapical granuloma undergoing cystic change.
 3. Epithelium proliferates and later covers the bare connective tissue surface of an abscess cavity or a cavity which may occur as a result of connective tissue breakdown by proteolytic enzyme activity.

12. Can inflammation occur in developmental cyst?

Ans. Yes, sometimes secondary inflammation can occur in developmental cysts.

ODONTOGENIC TUMORS

1. Define neoplasm, hamartoma and choristoma.

Ans. Hamartoma represents a dysmorphic proliferation of tissue that is native to the area and does not have the capacity for continuous growth but merely parallels that of the host.

 Examples: Odontome, AOT, hemangioma. Choristoma are similar to hamartomas except that they are dysmorphic proliferations of tissue that are not native to the site.

 Examples: A neoplasm can be defined as an abnormal mass of tissue, the growth of which exceeds and is uncoordinated with that of the normal tissues and persists in the same excessive manner after cessation of the stimuli which evoked the change (Willis 1952). Neoplasms may be 'Benign' or 'Malignant '.

 Examples: Benign—ameloblastoma, CEOT, fibroma, etc.
 Malignant—OSCC, verrucous carcinoma.

2. Which are locally aggressive odontogenic tumor?

Ans. • Ameloblastoma
• CEOT
• Odontogenic myxoma.

3. Different types of ameloblastoma.

Ans. • According to WHO 2005
• Unicystic ameloblastoma
• Solid/multicystic ameloblastoma
• Desmoplastic ameloblastoma
• Peripheral ameloblastoma
• According to WHO 2017
• Ameloblastoma, unicystic type
• Ameloblastoma, extraosseous/peripheral type
• Metastasizing ameloblastoma.

4. Histopathological variant of ameloblastoma.

Ans. Different histopathological variant of ameloblastoma are:
• Follicular ameloblastoma
• Plexiform ameloblastoma
• Desmoplastic ameloblastoma
• Granular ameloblastoma
• Acanthomatous ameloblastoma
• Keratoameloblastoma
• Hemangiomatous
• Basal cell ameloblastoma.

5. Is odontome a tumor, hamartoma or supernumerary tooth.

Ans. Some authors consider it as tumor, some as hamartoma and some as supernumerary tooth (compound odontome).

6. What are the different names of AOT?

Ans. 1. Adenoameloblastoma,
2. 2/3rd tumor as
2/3rd cases occur in anterior maxilla,
2/3rd cases are associated with impacted canine,
2/3rd are seen in females.

7. Different types of material and calcification seen in AOT?

Ans. Different types of material and calcification seen in AOT are:
• Enameloid
• Dentinoid
• Amyloid
• Basal lamina like
• Dystrophic calcification.

8. What are ghost cells, their pathogenesis and where they are seen?

Ans. The ghost cells are enlarged, ballooned, ovoid or elongated, elliptoid epithelial cells. They are eosinophlic and are usually well-defined, they may sometimes be blurred, and hence groups of them appear as fused. These epithelial cells are devoid of nuclei and they retain their basic cell outline.

Example of other cells without nucleus are RBCs, platelets.

Pathogenesis of ghost cell: Various theories has been given to explain the pathogenesis of ghost cell formation like:

- Aberrant keratinization
- Abnormal enamel matrix formation
- Local hypoxia and degeneration
- Coagulative necrosis
- Metaplasia of odontogenic epithelium
- Abnormal terminal differentiation or apoptosis
- Ghost cells are seen in calcifying odontogenic cyst, dentinogenic ghost cell tumor, odontome, odontoameloblastoma, etc.

9. Different types of material and calcified structure seen in CEOT.

Ans.
- Amyloid like material
  - Leisgang ring
  - Dystrophic calcification.

10. Why odontogenic myxoma has high recurrence potential?

Ans. The reason for high recurrence rates in odontogenic myxoma can be attributed to the local invasion of neoplasms between cancellous bone beyond radiographically visible margins and the lack of encapsulation. The production of mucoid ground substance is believed to be the cause for its growth, because increased mitotic activity and high proliferative rate are absent.

SALIVARY GLAND LESIONS

1. What are luminal and abluminal cells?

Ans. Luminal cells are the cells which lines the lumen of acini and duct, whereas abluminal cells are those which are away from lumen.

Examples luminal cells are serous and mucous cells. Lining cell of ducts.

Abluminal cells are basal cell of ducts and myoepithelial cells.

2. What is pleomorphic adenoma? Why it is called so?

Ans. Pleomorphic adenoma is benign epithelial tumor, also known as mixed tumor. The term mixed tumor of salivary gland does not imply origin from cells of more than one germ layer, it is simply used as a descriptive term for a neoplasm that characteristically showed combined features of epitheloid and connective tissue origin. Thus, the term is a misnomer. Also basic tumor pattern is highly variable, rarely are the individual tumor cells highly pleomorphic.

3. Where Swiss cheese pattern is seen?

Ans. Swiss cheese pattern is seen adenoid cystic carcinoma. It is the histopathological appearance.

4. Enumerate salivary gland tumor with nerve tissue propensity.

Ans. Adenoid cystic carcinoma and polymorphous low grade adenocarcinoma.

5. What are oncocytes?

Ans. An oncocyte is an epithelial cell characterized by an excessive number of mitochondria, resulting in an abundant acidophilic, granular cytoplasm. Oncocytes can be benign or malignant.

6. Chocolate color fluid seen in which salivary gland tumor?

Ans. Chocolate color fluid is seen in Warthin's tumor.

7. Cartilage seen in pleomorphic adenoma is true or false.

Ans. Cartilage seen in PA is pseudocartilage. It appear cartilaginous because of vacuolar degeneration of myoepithelial cells.

8. What are the different source of origin for intraosseous salivary gland tumor?

Ans. Different source of origin of MEC:
- Entrapment of retromolar mucous glands within the mandible.
- Developmentally included embryonic remnants of the submaxillary gland within the mandible.
- Neoplastic transformation of the mucous secreting cells found in the pluripotential epithelial lining of usually dentigerous cysts and other odontogenic cysts.
- Neoplastic transformation and invasion from the lining of the maxillary sinus.

REACTIVE LESIONS OF THE ORAL CAVITY

1. What is epulis?

Ans. Any localized gingival on gingiva is called epulis.

2. What are different types of fibroma?

Ans. Depending upon the cellularity (fibroblast) histopathologically termed acellular/hypocellular or cellular/hypercellular fibroma. But both the terms are misnomer and better terms are hypocellular and hypercellular fibroma. As there can be no collagen without cells (fibroblast).

3. What is peripheral cemento-ossifying fibroma?

Ans. It is a reactive lesion thought to arise from periodontal ligament and not the peripheral counter part of central ossifying fibroma. Histopathologically, it shows high degree of cellularity with bone formation, occasionally cementum-like material and dystrophic calcification.

4. Enumerate conditions and lesions causing gingival enlargement.

Ans. Gingival enlargement can be classified according to etiologic factors and pathologic changes as follows:

I. Inflammatory enlargement
   a. Chronic
   b. Acute

II. Drug-induced enlargement
   a. Anticonvulsants
   b. Immunosuppressants
   c. Calcium channel blockers

III. Enlargements associated with systemic diseases or conditions
   a. Conditioned enlargement
   1. Pregnancy
   2. Puberty
   3. Vitamin C deficiency
   4. Plasma cell gingivitis
   5. Nonspecific conditioned enlargement (pyogenic granuloma)
   b. Systemic diseases that cause gingival enlargement
   1. Leukemia
   2. Granulomatous diseases (e.g. Wegener's granulomatosis, sarcoidosis)
IV. Neoplastic enlargement (gingival tumors)
   a. Benign tumors
   b. Malignant tumors
V. False enlargement.

5. What are the different names for PGCG? Why term reparative granuloma is removed?

Ans. Other names for PGCG are as peripheral giant cell tumor, giant cell epulis, osteoclastoma, reparatory giant cell reparative granuloma, and giant cell hyperplasia of the oral mucosa, myeloid epulis and myeloid sarcoma. Initially, it was thought to be a reparative process but later on found that it is not a reparative rather a destructive lesion so term reparative was dropped.

6. What is the difference between granulation tissue and granuloma?

Ans. Granulation tissue is physiological seen during healing while granuloma is a pathological entity.

GIANT CELL LESIONS

1. What are giant cell? How they are formed?

Ans. Different theories has been put forward to explain the formation of giant cells:
- Division of monocyte/macrophage without cytoplasmic division
- More than one macrophage engulfing the same pathogen at same point of time
- Virally induced fusion of cells, e.g. EBV in lymphoma
- New macrophages engulf the old macrophage.

2. Classification of giant cells.

Ans. Giant cells are classified as physiological and pathological.

   Examples of physiological giant cells are osteoclasts in the bones, trophoblasts in placenta, megakaryocytes in the bone marrow.

   Examples of pathological giant cells are foreign body giant cells, Langhan's giant cells, Touton type giant cell, anaplastic tumor giant cell and Reed-Sternberg cell.

3. Lesion showing giant cell/enumerate giant cell lesion.

Ans. Lesion showing giant cells are:
   Classification
   1. Microbial lesions
      a. Tuberculosis
      b. Leprosy
      c. Actinomycosis

2. Tumor and tumor like lesion
   a. Central giant cell granuloma
   b. Peripheral giant cell granuloma
   c. Giant cell fibroma
   d. Osteosarcoma
   e. Rhabdomyosarcoma
   f. Hodgkin's lymphoma
3. Cystic lesion
   a. Traumatic bone cyst
   b. Aneurysmal bone cyst
4. Metabolic lesion: Hyperparathyroidism
5. Osteodystrophic lesion: Noonan-like multiple giant cell lesion syndrome
6. Miscellaneous lesion
   a. Cherubism
   b. Paget's disease
   c. Fibrous dysplasia.

4. Define osteomyelitis.

Ans. Osteomyelitis is an 'inflammatory condition of bone that begins as an infection of the medullary cavity and haversian system and extends to involve the periosteum of the affected area.'

5. What is sequestrum and involcrum?

Ans. • Sequestrum is dead necrotic bone
    • Involcrum is new bone formed.

FIBRO-OSSEOUS LESIONS

1. Define fibro-osseous lesions.

Ans. The term fibro-osseous lesion (FOL) is a generic designation of a group of jaw disorders characterized by the replacement of bone by a benign connective tissue matrix. This matrix displays varying degrees of mineralization in the form of woven bone or of cementum-like round acellular intensely basophilic structures.

2. Difference between ossifying fibroma and fibrous dysplasia.

Ans.

Fibrous dysplasia	Ossifying fibroma
Worth's concept: Disease of the bone	Disease within the bone
Etiology—genetic mutation—Gs alpha mutation	Unknown
Failure to reach a maturative stage of lamellar bone	Stimulation of undifferentiated mesenchymal stem cells
Single or multiple bones involved depending on the type	Single bone involved
Aggressive variety is less aggressive than aggressive variety of OF	Aggressive variety is more aggressive than aggressive variety of FD
Do not show root divergence and resorption	Resorption of roots occurs

3. Different calcified structure seen in FO lesion.

Ans. Osseous tissue, cementum like calcification and dystrophic calcification.

4. Syndrome associated with fibro-osseous lesions.

Ans. • Various syndrome associated with fibro-osseous lesion
- Jaffe's type polyostotic FD + skin pigmentation
- McCune Albright polyostotic FD + skin pigmentation
- Mazabraud's syndrome FD + intramuscular myxomas.

5. In which fibro-osseous lesion prominent resting and reversal line are seen?

Ans. In paget's disease prominent resting and reversal lines are seen.

6. What is Cherubism?

Ans. Also called multilocular cystic disease of the jaws. Term 'cherubism' because 'the full round cheeks and the upward cast of the eyes give the children a peculiarly' cherubic appearance. It is a symmetrical, multilocular, expansile radiolucent lesions of the mandible and/or the maxilla that typically first appear at the age of 2 to 7 years.

7. What do you mean by cafe au lait pigmentation? Name few lesions where it is seen?

Ans. Cafe au lait pigmentation means coffee mixed with milk appearance. Seen in fibrous dysplasia (irregular borders) and neurofibromatosis (regular borders).

TUMORS OF ORAL CAVITY

1. Define precancerous lesions and conditions. What is the new terminology used now?

Ans. World health organization (WHO) defined precancerous lesion as 'a morphologically altered tissue in which cancer is more likely to occur than in its apparently normal counterpart.' The precancerous condition in its turn is a generalized state associated with a significantly increased risk of cancer now the terminology used is oral potentially malignant disorder (OPMD).

2. Define leukoplakia. Enumerate different type of leukoplakia.

Ans. WHO 2005 defines it as 'a white plaque of questionable risk having excluded other known diseases or disorders that carry no increased risk of cancer'.

Type of leukoplakia are:
- Homogenous leukoplakia or heterogenous leukoplakia
- Proliferative verrucous leukoplakia
- Nodular/speckled leukoplakia
- Chronic hyperplastic leukoplakia.

3. Why verrucous carcinoma is misnomer?

Ans. Verrucous carcinoma has few but not all of the characteristics of a conventional malignancy (exhibiting progressive local growth and extension into underlying tissue, but lacking significant nuclear atypia and metastatic potential). Also there is no break in basement membrane which is defining feature of carcinoma. Therefore some authors are of view that word 'verrucous acanthosis' is a better substitute for this pathology.

4. Why term oral submucous fibrosis (OSMF) is misnomer?

Ans. Term OSMF denotes fibrosis of only submucosa and signifies lamina propria is spared. However OSMF is characterized by juxtaepithelial inflammation and progressive fibrosis of lamina propria and submucosa.

5. Where you see widening of PDL space?

Ans. Widening of PDL space is seen in osteosarcoma and scleroderma.

6. What are koilocytes?

Ans. Koilocytes are the virally (HPV) altered epithelial cells with perinuclear clear spaces and nuclear pyknosis.

7. Define dysplasia.

Ans. Term 'dys' mean abnormal and 'plasia' means formation.

Cytological and architectural features of oral epithelial dysplasia	
Cellular changes (atypia)	**Architectural (tissue) changes**
Abnormal variation in nuclear size (anisonucleosis)	Irregular epithelial stratification
Abnormal variation in nuclear shape (nuclear pleomorphism)	Loss of polarity of basal cells
Abnormal variation in cell size (anisocytosis)	Drop-shaped rete ridges
Abnormal variation in cell shape (cellular pleomorphism)	Increased number of mitotic figures
Increased nuclear-cytoplasmic ratio	Abnormally superficial mitoses
Increased nuclear size (dyskeratosis)	Premature keratinization in single cells
Atypical mitotic figures	Keratin pearls within rete pegs.
Increased number and size of nucleoli	

8. Lipoma salient features.

Ans. • Tissue specimen
   • Yellowish in color
   • Floats when put in formalin
   • Histopathologically shows signet ring appearance of fat cells.

9. What is exostosis, tori and osteoma?

Ans. • Exostoses are localized bony protuberances. Tori is an example of exostosis.
   • Osteoma is benign osteoblastic (bone forming) tumor.

10. Herring bone pattern seen in.

Ans. Fibrosarcoma.

11. Define oral lichen planus.

Ans. Lichen planus is an autoimmune mucocutaneous disorder in which oral involvement precedes the appearance of other symptoms or lesions at other locations. It is defined by Erasmus Wilson as eruption of pimples remarkable for their color, their figure, their structure, their habits of isolated and aggregated development, their habitat, their local and chronic character and for the melasmic stains which they leave behind them when they disappear.

12. Enumerate the characteristic features seen in oral lichen planus.

Ans. Characteristic features seen in oral lichen planus:

   Clinically
   • Wickham's striae
   • Bilateral presentation

Histopathologically
- Civatte, hyaline, cytoid bodies
- Max-Joseph spaces
- Basal cell degeneration
- Liquefactive degeneration of basement membrane subepithelial band of chronic inflammatory cells infiltrate.

13. Define neoplasm.

Ans. A neoplasm can be defined as an abnormal mass of tissue, the growth of which exceeds and is uncoordinated with that of the normal tissues and persists in the same excessive manner after cessation of the stimuli which evoked the change (Willis 1952).

DENTAL CARIES AND PULPAL PATHOLOGIES

1. Define dental caries?

Ans. Dental caries is an irreversible polymicrobial disease of the calcified tissues of the teeth, characterized by demineralization of the inorganic portion and destruction of the organic substance of the tooth, which often leads to cavitations. The word caries is derived from the Latin word meaning 'rot' or 'decay'.

2. What are different theories for etiology of dental caries?

Ans. Different theories for caries etiology are:
- The legend of worms
- Endogenous theories
- Chemical theory
- Parasitic theory
- Miller's chemico-parasitic theory or the acidogenic theory
- Proteolytic theory
- The proteolysis chelation theory.

3. What is liquefaction foci of Miller?

Ans. Bacteria penetrate the dentinal tubules and gives beaded appearance on decalcified section. Bacteria produce acids which cause breakdown of dentinal tubules and formation of foci of Miller. 'Liquefaction foci' are formed by focal coalescence and breakdown of a w dentinal tubules.

4. What is pulpitis and its types?

Ans. Inflammation of pulp is called pulpitis. Different type of pulpitis are:
- Acute or chronic pulpitis
- Chronic hyperplastic pulpitis
- Reversible or irreversible pulpitis
- First change seen in pulpitis is pulpal hyperemia.

5. What is wheatsheafing of odontoblast?

Ans. Due to pulpitis there is hydropic degeneration of odontoblast. This may affect either individual cells or group of adjacent cells to produce spherical foci of localized liquefaction within the odontoblast layer. These globules of fluid squeeze together the intervening group of odontoblast so that they become elongated, while their midportion is compressed to form waist like indentations giving 'wheatsheafing' appearance.

6. Enumerate different types of calcification seen in pulp and their pathogenesis.

Ans. Different type of calcification seen in pulp are:

- Denticles (pulp stone).
- True pulp stone (contain dentinal tubules).
- False pulp stone (without dentinal tubules).
- Diffuse calcification.
- Denticles are mostly seen in pulp chamber and diffuse calcification seen in root canals.
- Diffuse calcification are formed due to aging. With aging secondary dentin forms leading to decrease in size of pulp space. Also with aging fibrosis occur. This leads to deposition of minerals upon the fibers leading to diffuse calcification.
- False pulp stone formation occur due to deposition of minerals upon the nidus. Nidus is mainly in the form of degenerated cells and damaged blood vessels. Calcification of blood vessel is called atherosclerosis.
- True pulp stone are the stone which contain dentinal tubules. They follow the physiological process of normal odontogenesis. During odontogenesis some epithelial cells get entrapped in the pulpal tissue, which later on get activated by a stimulus. Upon activation epithelial cell induce dental mesenchymal cells to transform into odontoblast, leading to formation of true stone.
- Some state that enamel proteins embedded during development of tooth act as signalling to mesenchymal pulpal cell to form odontoblast leading to formation of true pulp stone.

MISCELLANEOUS

1. Enumerate different types of Candida.

Ans. Candidiasis is a fungal infection caused by candidia. Different Candida species are *C. albicans, C. krusei, C. tropicalis. C. parapsilosis,* etc.

Different types of candida infection are:

- Acute form
- Pseudomembranous candidiasis (oral thrush)
- Erythematous
- Chronic form
- Hyperplastic (candidal leukoplakia)
- Nodular
- Plaque like
- Erythematous
- Pseudomembranous
- Candida associated lesions
- Denture stomatitis (chronic atrophic candidiasis)
- Angular cheilitis
- Median rhomboid glossitis.

2. Why oral hairy leukoplakia (OHL) is a misnomer?

Ans. OHL is an asymptomatic white lesion on the lateral border of the tongue, unilaterally or bilaterally, with indefinite boundaries and a flat, corrugated or hairy surface, that is not removable on scraping. Leukoplakia is diagnosis of exclusion. The term 'hairy leukoplakia' is therefore, misleading as it is a definable lesion. Furthermore, the lesion is not premalignant in nature.

3. What is Greenspan lesion and Grinspan syndrome?

Ans. Greenspan lesion is oral hairy leukoplakia. Grinspan syndrome is associated with oral lichen planus (OLP). It is triad of OLP, diabetes mellitus and hypertension.

4. Why infectious mononucleosis term is misnomer?

Ans. Infectious mononucleosis (IM) is an infection commonly caused by the Epstein-Barr virus. In IM some of the lymphocytes will be extremely large, mimicking monocytes, hence the term mononucleosis is used which is a misnomer because the cells are actually altered lymphocytes. Some will appear atypical which is a hallmark of the disease. A 50% absolute lymphocytosis with 10% atypical lymphocytes is diagnostic.

5. Where you see Lipschütz bodies and Anitschkow cells?

Ans. Lipschütz bodies are seen in herpes simplex infection. These are intranuclear inclusions bodies. Anitschkow cells are seen in recurrent aphthous ulcer, sickle cell disease, megaloblastic anemias, and iron-deficiency anemias, in children receiving chemotherapy for cancer, and even in normal people. Anitschkow cells elongated nuclei containing a linear bar of chromatin with radiating processes of chromatin extending towards the nuclear membrane.

6. Why is the term 'agranulocytosis' a misnomer?

Ans. Agranulocytosis means increase in agranulocytes. However, there is decrease in number of granulocytes and because of this there is relative increase in agranulocytes in comparison to granulocytes.

7. Define pus.

Ans. A thick, whitish-yellow fluid that results from the accumulation of white blood cells, liquefied tissue, and cellular debris. Pus is commonly a sign of infection or foreign material in the body. Localized collection of pus is called abscess.

Recommended Further Reading

1. Reichart PA, Philipsen HP. Odontogenic tumors and allied lesions. London: Quintessence Publishing Co Ltd.; 2004.
2. Spouge JD. Oral pathology. St Louis: MO, CV Mosby; 1973.
3. Rajendran R, Sivapathasundharam B. Shafers' textbook of Oral Pathology. 7th ed. New Delhi, India: Elsevier; 2012.
4. Neville BW, Damm DD, Allen CM, Bouquot JE. Oral and Maxillofacial Pathology. 3rd ed. India: Elsevier; 2013.
5. Shear M, Speight P. Cysts of the Oral and Maxillofacial Regions. 4th ed. Oxford: Blackwell Munksgaard; 2007.
6. Bafna SS, Joy T, Tupkari JV, Landge JS. Dentinogenic ghost cell tumor. J Oral Maxillofac Pathol. 2016;20:163.
7. Thakur A, Tupkari JV, Joy T, Jugade SC, Chellappa N. Keratocystic odontogenic tumour - An unusual presentation. J Oral Med, Oral Surg, Oral Pathol, Oral Radiol. 2017; 3(4): 225–7.
8. Khurana D, Thakur A, Kadam A, Tupkari JV. Desmoplastic Ameloblastoma-An unusual presentation. J Oral Med, Oral Surg, Oral Pathol, Oral Radiol. 2017; 3(3):172–5.
9. Thakur A, Tupkari JV, Wadde KR, Patil M, Alam N. Tubercular osteomyelitis of the mandible– A case report. J Oral Med, Oral Surg, Oral Pathol, Oral Radiol. 2017; 3(4): 228–30.
10. Joy TC, Bafna S, Tupkari JV, Ahire M. Cysts of the orofacial region: A 35 year demographic data at an Indian dental institute. Int J Adv Res. 2017;5:24–41.